Donna Vallone

How Wealth Links to Health

Donna Vallone

How Wealth Links to Health

Testing Theories to Explain Socioeconomic Disparities in Disease and Death

VDM Verlag Dr. Müller

Impressum/Imprint (nur für Deutschland/ only for Germany)
Bibliografische Information der Deutschen Nationalbibliothek: Die Deutsche Nationalbibliothek
verzeichnet diese Publikation in der Deutschen Nationalbibliografie; detaillierte bibliografische
Daten sind im Internet über http://dnb.d-nb.de abrufbar.
Alle in diesem Buch genannten Marken und Produktnamen unterliegen warenzeichen-, marken-
oder patentrechtlichem Schutz bzw. sind Warenzeichen oder eingetragene Warenzeichen der
jeweiligen Inhaber. Die Wiedergabe von Marken, Produktnamen, Gebrauchsnamen,
Handelsnamen, Warenbezeichnungen u.s.w. in diesem Werk berechtigt auch ohne besondere
Kennzeichnung nicht zu der Annahme, dass solche Namen im Sinne der Warenzeichen- und
Markenschutzgesetzgebung als frei zu betrachten wären und daher von jedermann benutzt
werden dürften.

Coverbild: www.purestockx.com

Verlag: VDM Verlag Dr. Müller Aktiengesellschaft & Co. KG
Dudweiler Landstr. 125 a, 66123 Saarbrücken, Deutschland
Telefon +49 681 9100-698, Telefax +49 681 9100-988, Email: info@vdm-verlag.de
Zugl.: New York, Columbia University, Diss., 2003

Herstellung in Deutschland:
Schaltungsdienst Lange o.H.G., Zehrensdorfer Str. 11, D-12277 Berlin
Books on Demand GmbH, Gutenbergring 53, D-22848 Norderstedt
Reha GmbH, Dudweiler Landstr. 99, D- 66123 Saarbrücken
ISBN: 978-3-639-07902-9

Imprint (only for USA, GB)
Bibliographic information published by the Deutsche Nationalbibliothek: The Deutsche
Nationalbibliothek lists this publication in the Deutsche Nationalbibliografie; detailed
bibliographic data are available in the Internet at http://dnb.d-nb.de.
Any brand names and product names mentioned in this book are subject to trademark, brand or
patent protection and are trademarks or registered trademarks of their respective holders. The use
of brand names, product names, common names, trade names, product descriptions etc. even
without
a particular marking in this works is in no way to be construed to mean that such names may be
regarded as unrestricted in respect of trademark and brand protection legislation and could thus
be used by anyone.

Cover image: www.purestockx.com

Publisher:
VDM Verlag Dr. Müller Aktiengesellschaft & Co. KG
Dudweiler Landstr. 125 a, 66123 Saarbrücken, Germany
Phone +49 681 9100-698, Fax +49 681 9100-988, Email: info@vdm-verlag.de

Copyright © 2008 VDM Verlag Dr. Müller Aktiengesellschaft & Co. KG and licensors
All rights reserved. Saarbrücken 2008

Produced in USA and UK by:
Lightning Source Inc., 1246 Heil Quaker Blvd., La Vergne, TN 37086, USA
Lightning Source UK Ltd., Chapter House, Pitfield, Kiln Farm, Milton Keynes, MK11 3LW, GB
BookSurge, 7290 B. Investment Drive, North Charleston, SC 29418, USA
ISBN: 978-3-639-07902-9

TABLE OF CONTENTS

LIST OF TABLES AND FIGURES

Chapter I

Introduction

Do people have worse health because they are "relatively deprived"—dissatisfied, frustrated, humiliated, and stressed out because of where they stand relative to others in their communities, or is their worse health due to the fact that they are materially disadvantaged with respect to health-related resources? For example, do those at the top of the income structure within Washington Heights experience better health outcomes than those at the bottom of the Upper West Side, or do absolute resources translate across place and position to influence health and longevity? Both perspectives have been put forth to explain the persistence of the graded association between health and wealth, particularly within industrialized societies where the majority of the population is not considered poor. While evidence has been marshaled for both perspectives, direct tests of the competing ideas are extremely rare.

SES Differentials in Morbidity and Mortality

While there is little question that socioeconomic status (SES) is a strong and pervasive predictor of health status and life expectancy, persisting across time and place (Chapin 1924; Coombs 1941; Kitagawa and Hauser 1973; Pappas et al. 1993; Williams and Collins 1995; Coombs 1941; Kitagawa and Hauser 1973; Pappas et al. 1993; Williams and Collins 1995), the causal mechanisms behind the association remain poorly understood. As early as the 19th century, reports that people at the top of the socioeconomic ladder were living healthier and longer began to emerge (Chadwick 1842). Although mortality rates have decreased and life expectancy has increased over the last century, disparities in health and longevity are invariably related to differences in wealth (Feinstein 1993). Generally, the time at which one dies is related to one's SES (Antonovsky 1967), and the wealthy are healthier and tend to live longer (Evans 1994).

The magnitude and persistence of the association between SES, health status and mortality give rise to complex and important questions about the determinants of health and longevity, particularly within the developed nations of the world. Although SES patterns of disease and death have been repeatedly documented since the mid-1800s, theories to explain how SES operates remain controversial.

Much of the early research linking socioeconomic status to health and life expectancy began in Britain, a result of British death certificates being coded with social or occupational class categories. Prior to 1980, many in Britain assumed that progressive policies in terms of employment, housing, and welfare services would serve to reduce class-based health inequalities (Wilkinson 1986b). A general consensus presumed that improvements in social welfare would inevitably result in health equity across socioeconomic status. However, investigators using census data found standardized mortality rates for all causes of death decreased at each of six increasing occupational status levels (Adelstein 1980). In 1982, a British government report, commonly known as the Black Report, released findings of increasing mortality inequalities between occupational class groups (Black et al. 1982). Although the study was criticized for its use of cross-sectional decennial census information, and calculating mortality rates using denominators based on death certificate occupational status, it stimulated an interest in further examining SES morbidity and mortality differentials.

Researchers embarked on overcoming the limitations of cross-sectional analyses by conducting large-scale, longitudinal studies. In 1984, the landmark Whitehall study, which followed over ten thousand British civil servants, found that the age-standardized mortality, over a ten-year period, among males aged forty to sixty-four, was over three times as high for those in clerical and manual grades as in the senior administrative positions (Marmot, Shipley, and Rose 1984). In addition, findings indicated gradations in mortality at each level of the social hierarchy. Mortality rates varied continuously and precisely with the individual's civil service grade, suggesting that differences in mortality were linked to factors other than abject poverty. While the Whitehall study civil service status groupings reflected differences in income and status of position, all respondents were employed and receiving British national health insurance. This SES-mortality gradient has also been found in US studies. Kitagawa and Hauser (1973) found that an increase in years of education was associated with a lower risk of death. More recently, Pappas and his colleagues found a graded association between mortality and both income and education (Pappas et al. 1993). It has been found that individuals in families with incomes greater than $50,000 in 1980 had a life expectancy about 25 percent longer than those in families with incomes less than $5,000 (Rogot, Sorlie, and Johnson 1992). Social gradients in morbidity, comparable to the British findings, have been demonstrated with many of the large survey data collections such as the Wisconsin Longitudinal Study of 1958 high school graduates, and the US National Survey of Families and Households (Marmot et al. 1997). Given the challenges associated with being poor and undereducated, it is not surprising that material deprivation should be related to ill health and untimely death. However, findings indicate that differences in morbidity and mortality exist along a finely stratified continuum of SES such that the risk of dying increases almost threefold between the bottom and the top of the social ladder (Sorlie, Backlund, and Keller 1995) (Evans 1994).

This graded relationship suggests that some SES-related processes are not only operating on those who are impoverished, unemployed, or without access to health care, but on the entire population to a greater or lesser degree. Furthermore, findings indicate that declines in mortality rates in 1986 were substantially greater for those at the top of the hierarchy than in 1960, suggesting mortality differentials may be increasing over time (Pappas et al. 1993). The idea that the mid-level manager in a one-bedroom apartment faces worse health outcomes than his boss in the three-bedroom duplex on the other side of town has prompted researchers all over the world to try to explain this phenomenon (Goode 1999).

Psychosocial and Materialist Perspectives

Several hypotheses have been put forth to explain mortality and morbidity differentials in relation to SES. Historically, explanations have fallen into two broad categories, social selection and social causation. Social selection explanations involve two processes, one in which health directly affects SES by limiting the acquisition of education, income and occupational position, and the second in which pre-existing attributes such as IQ and height affect both social position and health, and thereby, explain the links from SES to health. This approach indicates that the healthier rise up on the social hierarchy and the less healthy move downward. Alternatively, social causation frameworks posit that different social environments causally influence health. Following a decade of empirical research and debate, there is some consensus that genetics, social selection, and access to health care services explains only a portion of the SES variation in health (Bartley and Plewis 1997) (Evans 1994). Social causation theories that view social conditions as causally related to health outcomes have gained ascendancy.

3

While strides in reducing or preventing infectious and chronic disease have led to increased life expectancy, the influence of social conditions on health status and survival has remained relatively stable or has increased (Hummer, Rogers, and Eberstein 1998; Link and Phelan 1995; Pappas et al. 1993). To explain the SES-health gradient, especially within industrialized populations where abject poverty is relatively absent, some researchers have focused on examining psychosocial processes related to social position. Adler's seminal paper, "The Challenge of the Gradient," reviewed empirical evidence concerning the SES-health relationship, and theorized that psychosocial processes are critical for understanding the connection between SES and health. Among other things, Adler and colleagues suggested that psychological stress, engendered as a result of one's position within the hierarchy, might affect the nervous system so as to increase one's susceptibility to disease, thus, increasing morbidity and mortality (Adler et al. 1994).

Wilkinson and others took this idea of hierarchical stress a step further. Stemming from an interpretation of the epidemiological transition, a stage in economic development after which further improvements in material standards have less influence on health, Wilkinson suggested that health inequalities reflect the direct and indirect psychosocial effects of income inequality (Wilkinson 1996). Greater inequality in income distribution is theorized to generate relative deprivation, a constellation of feelings of inadequacy deriving from one's relative position within the social hierarchy (Wilkinson 1997a; Jones and Sidell 1997; Jones and Sidell 1997). According to Wilkinson, this process occurs irrespective of the absolute income level of countries. Wilkinson claims support for this theory in the finding that nations with large income disparities experience worse health outcomes than those with lower income disparities, despite adjustment for average income level and GNP (Wilkinson 1986a; Wilkinson 1986b; Wilkinson 1992; Wilkinson 1996; Wilkinson 1986b; Wilkinson 1992; Wilkinson 1996). Wilkinson also cites the differences in health status between US states in relation to levels of income inequality as further evidence for his hypothesis.

Early findings of the cross-sectional association between income inequality and life expectancy stimulated enthusiasm among researchers interested in explaining health inequalities around the world. Numerous studies have investigated income inequality at different levels of geographical aggregation, using a variety of measures of income dispersion. However, findings

4

confirming the nature of the relationship between income inequality and health outcomes have so far proved inconclusive.

According to Wilkinson (1997b), "...socioeconomic differences in health within countries result primarily from differences in people's position in the socioeconomic hierarchy relative to others, leaving a less powerful role to the undoubted direct effects of absolute material standards." Negative psychosocial injuries deriving from deprivation, whether objective or subjective, are well documented (Sennett and Cobb 1973), and have been found to affect health (Syme and Berkman 1976; Thoits 1995; Thoits 1995). However, questions remain concerning the prevalence of social comparison processes such as relative deprivation (Mirowsky 1987), and the contribution of such psychosocial factors in explaining the SES-health relationship. While Wilkinson has argued about the primacy of psychosocial processes such as relative deprivation in explaining health inequalities within countries (Wilkinson 1997b), relative deprivation, the underlying mechanism theorized to explain the relationship between income inequality and health outcomes, has not been empirically examined within the context of the income inequality debate.

Some suggest that this perspective seeks to separate psychological processes from the material conditions embedded in everyday life. Critics suggest that this explanation decontextualizes psychosocial effects from its structural origins, which establishes stratification (Lynch et al. 2000). With respect to attitudes of deprivation, investigators in the area of social justice research have found that a majority of the population in western societies considers their share of material goods "just," while only a minority indicated that they were "underpaid" or "unsatisfied" with their income level (Wegener 1991). Thus, social comparison processes such as relative deprivation based on income levels may exist for a relatively small portion of the population. While stress, regardless of origin, has been associated with poor health outcomes (Thoits 1995), the role of stress deriving from position within the social order has not been adequately examined.

Alternatively, explanations that emphasize the conditions under which people experience their daily lives have been termed "materialist perspectives." According to these explanations, health inequalities derive from structural processes that differentially distribute material resources within a society. House and his colleagues began to formulate materialist explanations for SES health disparities in their work on aging, health and social class (House et al. 1990).

5

They asserted that an individual's current, past and future experiences are determined by their position within the social stratification system (House et al. 1992). These experiences, which translate into patterns of social opportunities and barriers associated with statuses such as SES, race/ethnicity, age, and gender, are hypothesized to significantly define aspects of human health and functioning. Thus, SES differentials in health are a reflection of the stratification system itself.

Building on the work of House and his colleagues, Link and Phelan (1995) put forth a hypothesis, Fundamental Cause for Social Disparities in Disease and Death, to explain the process by which the SES-health relationship operates throughout the hierarchy. Their main premise rests on the claim that socioeconomic resources, rather than health risk behaviors, generate stratification in health status and life expectancy. Link and Phelan explain that resources in the form of knowledge, money, power, and social connections are utilized at every level of the social hierarchy to reduce risks and adopt protective strategies, regardless of the nature and pathway of health threats (Link et al. 1998). Their theory posits that as new health information and technology develops, those at the top of the SES hierarchy are always best positioned to benefit from advances in treatment and risk reduction strategies by virtue of their being able to leverage resources to employ them (Link and Phelan 1995).

Link and Phelan (2000) indicate that this dynamic process of utilizing resources operates to change the patterns of which specific diseases individuals are likely to experience and how long they live, while serving to maintain the relationship between SES, morbidity and mortality. For example, in the early part of the 20th century, those at the top of the socioeconomic ladder lived relatively sedentary lives and being overweight was considered to reflect a degree of wealth and comfort. During this time, risk for disease and death was largely due to infectious disease, resulting from a lack of sanitation and immunization. Today, chronic disease has replaced infectious disease as the most serious threat to health and longevity. As a result, characteristics such as being overweight and sedentarism are now considered intervening risk factors for several chronic conditions. According to Link and Phelan, such intervening mechanisms between SES and health are continually replaced in relation to the social patterns of disease (Link and Phelan 1996). This emergence of new risk factors that mediate the SES-health relationship serves to maintain this persistent association, even in the context of eradicating or reducing specific risk behaviors or conditions.

Their resource utilization argument describes a process that operates on several levels. On one level, the process weds the products of structural distribution systems such as money, knowledge, power and prestige to individual agency in that to the extent possible, people employ resources to promote health. At the same time, individuals with resources simply benefit from the context within which they live and work. For example, higher SES groups tend to be employed in organizations that offer health insurance coverage, and live in residential neighborhoods that are free of industrial pollutants. In effect, resource utilization can produce an "ecological effect" by conferring collective social health for resource-rich groups through a higher probability of experiencing healthy situations (Kaufman and Cooper 1999).

According to the Fundamental Cause explanation, SES reflects a portfolio of available resources, which are employed to reduce morbidity and mortality in an additive fashion at each level of the hierarchy, resulting in the finely stratified relationships between SES, health, and life expectancy. Those resources can be leveraged to help ease any negative life event in an infinite number of ways, regardless of the nature and complexity of the issue. On average, even a slight reduction in resource level constrains choices, resulting in increased risk of disease and death. Those with fewer resources than those above them, even in the upper income brackets, are always at some disadvantage in being able to reduce risk and engage in health-promoting behaviors.

Although Link and Phelan emphasize material processes to explain SES health disparities rather than psychosocial mechanisms, they indicate that the psychosocial perspective, which highlights hierarchical stress, is compatible with their hypothesis. Stress, regardless of its origin or form, can be considered one more health-related risk, which can be reduced or avoided by resource-rich individuals (Link and Phelan 2000). While Link and Phelan acknowledge the important role stress plays in increasing host vulnerability to disease processes, Fundamental Cause theory diverges from the hierarchy stress approach in that it attributes objective material conditions as the primary factor in explaining SES health differentials. According to Wilkinson, the social hierarchy is the constant that drives the persistent relationship between health and SES. Link et al. (1998) contend that the hierarchical stress hypothesis is limited in that it predicts a constant association between SES and stress-related diseases while in the case of coronary heart disease, the association has changed over the last several decades--- while it had been characterized as a "disease of the wealthy," those at the bottom of the hierarchy are now more likely to suffer from heart disease   Fundamental Cause theory shifts the emphasis from the consequences of stratification such as hierarchical stress, to an examination of the products of the social stratification system i.e. resources, and how they are utilized to establish and reproduce SES-related health inequalities.

While theories explaining the SES-health gradient remain controversial, the specific mechanisms proposed to explain how social conditions influence health require further empirical investigation. This work seeks to examine the characterization and relative importance of two proposed mechanisms by providing supporting evidence as to the whether material resources or psychosocial processes matter more in mediating the association between SES, health, and longevity. To that end, the available literature pertaining to these two theoretical perspectives will be reviewed to determine the strengths and the weaknesses of current empirical evidence in Chapter II. Chapter III introduces the dataset, the Health and Retirement Study, upon which all analyses will be conducted. In Chapter IV, the general analytic approach is outlined, and measurement issues related to all key variables are discussed. Chapters V and VI present the empirical findings related to the specific hypotheses of this study. Chapter VII concludes by summarizing the results, discussing the implications of the findings, and suggesting possible areas for further research.

Chapter II

Current Theoretical Perspectives and Relevant Research

A paradox inherent in the scientific method is that, attached though
we are to the hypotheses we formulate, we must really subject them to assault and search for
circumstances that really test their resilience
(Paneth and Susser 1995).

Debates concerning the SES-health gradient center on two important explanatory

mechanisms: materialist and psychosocial factors. At the core of the debate is the challenge of

explaining how socioeconomic status translates into different health outcomes, especially in the

context of the industrialized world. Although poverty continues to exist within the wealthiest of

nations such as the US, health disparities, most surprisingly, continue to persist at the middle and

upper income levels. The fundamental question of why this graded association continues to

persist has prompted researchers to look beyond the correlates of low income to how

socioeconomic status shapes experiences, and patterns of social factors or conditions, which in

effect, influence health outcomes.

Psychosocial Perspectives: Income Inequality and Relative Deprivation

In recent years, some investigators have focused on a related aspect of socioeconomic

status: income distribution, and how it relates to morbidity and mortality. This area of inquiry

began with Rodgers who conducted an international cross-sectional analysis of income

distribution and determinants of mortality among fifty-six (56) countries (Rodgers 1979).

Greater income inequality was found to be associated with higher mortality, suggesting that

income distribution, in addition to absolute income, may play an important role in explaining

health inequalities (Rodgers 1979). Several studies followed and produced similar results.

Waldmann reported a significant relationship between the proportion of the top 5% of the

household income distribution and infant mortality (Waldmann 1992). Wilkinson, the researcher

most associated with evidence and arguments for the income inequality hypothesis, found

evidence of a significant relationship between income distribution and mortality in contrast to a

weak association between average income as measured by gross national product per capita and

life expectancy among 23 countries within the Organization for Economic Cooperation and

Development (OECD) (Wilkinson 1992). To explain this finding, Wilkinson suggested that relative, rather than absolute income, explains the association between income distribution and health. This shift to relative standards reduces the significance of material circumstances and elevates the importance of psychosocial factors (Wilkinson 1992).

Results of numerous analyses have supported the hypothesis that greater income inequality negatively influences health. However, critics raised important methodological concerns regarding the empirical evidence (Judge 1995; Fiscella and Franks 1997; Gravelle 1998; Fiscella and Franks 1997; Gravelle 1998). Much of the concern focused on the quality and cross-sectional nature of the country-level data, the lack of control for potential confounding variables, the measurement of income inequality, and the inability to account for changes in income inequality over time. Judge (1995) argued that some of Wilkinson's data reflected comparisons of two different groups of countries across different time periods, and questioned Wilkinson's indicator of income inequality: family income. While Judge found support for the income inequality hypothesis when using the family income indicator, measures of income per capita did not reveal a similar finding, suggesting that the choice of indicator may influence the outcome. Others have suggested that the association might, at least in part, be due to a statistical artifact as a result of using population rather than individual data (Gravelle 1998). This argument draws upon the "ecological fallacy" which cautions epidemiologists against inferring from population-level correlations to individual risk estimates. In effect, the association between income inequality and mortality may represent confounding by family income at the individual level.

In response to these methodological criticisms, researchers set about to test the validity of the relationship between income inequality and health outcomes using individual-level longitudinal data, varying the measures of income inequality as well as the levels of geographic aggregation. Using 1980 and 1990 Census data for the less well-off 50% of the population, Kaplan and colleagues found no important correlation between 1980-1990 changes in US state income inequality and 1980-1990 trends in mortality. However, this ecological study was unable to control adequately for confounding and effect modification at the individual level.

Using two measures of income inequality, the Gini coefficient and the Robin Hood Index, Kennedy found them to be significantly associated with mortality, even after adjusting for poverty. However, the study's cross-sectional design limits the interpretation of these findings, and its use of ecological measures prevents generalizing to the individual level. In a study that

10

examined income inequality in 282 US metropolitan areas using three measures of income inequality and mortality, associations varied across inequality measures (Lynch et al. 1998). When identical analyses varied only the level of geographical aggregation from US county to census tract level, differences in effect size suggest that income inequality might also depend of level of aggregation (Soobader and LeClere 1999). Comparison of models also demonstrated the overestimation of the effect of income inequality when the individual-level socioeconomic variables were excluded, thereby highlighting the necessity to include all levels through which SES may operate to influence health (Soobader and LeClere 1999).

Researchers suggested that future analyses of income inequality and health need to link micro-level information to macro-level processes (Kaplan et al. 1996). In response, Fiscella and Franks examined the effect of inequality between communities (approximated US counties or combined county areas), independent of individually measured household income, on mortality in the United States. Although survival, adjusted for age, sex, family size, and mean community income, was associated with inequality, when family income was added into the model, the relationship was insignificant (Fiscella and Franks 1997). They concluded that many of the previous ecological analyses might have overstated the relationship between income distribution and health outcomes by not adequately controlling for the confounding of individual income.

Daly and colleagues used micro-level data that matched health status with aggregate-level inequality measures. Using mortality data from the 1980 and 1990 National Center for Health Statistics (NCHS) mortality files, state-level inequality from census data, and income and demographic data from the 1978 and 1988 Panel Study of Income Dynamics (PSID), state-level inequality measures in 1980 and 1990 were regressed on individual mortality risk over the five-year period surrounding the 1980 and 1990 censuses (Daly et al. 1998). All regressions controlled for age, race, sex, and median state income as well as for family size (which had no effect on the results). Although a subgroup analysis of middle-income non-elderly (25-64) individuals revealed a significant association between inequality and mortality, no effects of inequality on mortality risk on the full sample (25-65 plus) was found, and adjusting for individual income produced inconsistent results.

Kennedy et al. (1998) employed hierarchical linear modeling (HLM) to reduce misspecification and the attribution of a contextual effect when none exists. This analysis was conducted to determine the effects of state-level income inequality, as measured by the Gini

11

Coefficient, on self-rated health status, controlling for individual socioeconomic status (Kennedy, Kawachi, and Prothrow-Stith 1996). Age, educational attainment, health insurance status, household composition, race and household income were included in the various models. Individual-level data was obtained from the 1993 and 1994 Behavioral Risk Factor Surveillance System (BRFSS) surveys, a random-digit telephone survey designed to produce comparable state-level representation of the United States non-institutionalized population. In contrast to the results of Fiscella & Franks (1997) who found that the effect of income inequality at a community level disappeared when individual income was included in the model, Kennedy et al. (1998) found an independent effect for state-level inequality on health status after controlling for household income. Furthermore, the effect of inequality was present for those in the middle-income bracket (20-35K/yr). Kennedy and colleagues speculated that the divergent findings might have been the result of differing geographic levels of income inequality, and that Fiscella and Franks' analysis may have underestimated the effect of income inequality by using income distributions from each area's sample that were truncated at $25,000.

Diez-Roux and colleagues examined the relation between state-level income inequality and cardiovascular disease (CVD) risk factors (Diez-Roux, Link, and Northridge 2000). In an effort to disentangle individual and contextual effects, multi-level models were employed to determine whether group-level income inequality would be associated with risk factor levels (body mass index, hypertension, smoking and sedentarism), rather than the association be the result of confounding by individual-level income. Although positive associations of income inequality with risk factor levels were found to persist after controlling for individual-level income, associations did not persist across income levels. For example, body mass index and hypertension were negatively associated with income inequality at high-income levels, while sedentarism was positively associated at lower income levels. Smoking was positively associated with income inequality, but not at lower income levels. Although the findings suggest a contextual effect of income inequality on CVD risk factor levels, the authors were reluctant to draw definite conclusions.

While substantial evidence of an increase in income inequality in the United States has existed since the 1970s (Karoly 1993; Danziger and Gottschalk 1995), findings about the income inequality-health association remain unclear. In addition, the appropriate level of analysis is still a question. In a recent US study, investigators examined the association of income inequality

12

measured at three levels of geographic aggregation—state, metropolitan area (MA) and county levels on self-rated health using multi-level modeling techniques (Blakely, Lochner, and Kawachi 2002). Investigators found little overall association of county-level or metropolitan area income inequality with self-rated health, particularly when adjusting for individual-level income. State-level income inequality was found to be stronger for those within non-metropolitan areas (i.e., rural). Current research has not adequately determined whether income inequality influences population health at the neighborhood, county, city and other geographic levels (Veenstra 2002).

In a comprehensive re-examination of the empirical evidence regarding income inequality and population health, Mellor and Milyo (2001) found little consistent or strong evidence to support the income inequality hypothesis. They argue that the absence of controls for demographic differences across US states other than age, and the failure to control for longitudinal state-specific effects has resulted in spurious findings that have served to support the assertion of robust associations across US states (Mellor and Milyo 2001).

Wilkinson derived a theory to explain how income disparities might influence population health. Drawing upon the "epidemiological transition," defined as a shift in the major causes of death from infectious to chronic disease thought to be related to the economic development of a nation (Omran 1971), Wilkinson postulated that psychosocial consequences related to social position, rather than material circumstances, must be the key to explaining the gradient in health among those who are not poor (Wilkinson 1994). Wilkinson theorized that since societies fail to realize substantial health improvements as a result of increases in absolute material standards in the later stages of industrialization, relative deprivation resulting from income inequality is the causal mechanism through which SES affects health and longevity. Relative deprivation, defined as a constellation of feelings of inadequacy and discontent related to one's position within the social order, has been theorized to cause stress, manifesting in difficulties in maintaining social bonds, lack of self-esteem, shame, and distrust, thereby, affecting health (Elstad 1998). Stress related to social position, also known as hierarchical stress, is thought to operate through two pathways: directly by altering biological processes to reduce an individual's susceptibility to disease (Cassel 1976), and indirectly by causing individuals to engage in health-damaging behaviors (Wilkinson 1997b). Wilkinson concludes that psychosocial mechanisms related to social

13

position significantly explain health disparities, independent of material conditions and particularly within developed countries (Wilkinson 1997b; Wilkinson 1997a).

While relative deprivation is new to social epidemiology, Stouffer and colleagues first introduced the concept of relative deprivation more than 50 years ago in the seminal work, *The American Soldier* (Stouffer et al. 1949). In this large study of Army life during World War II, researchers were surprised to find that soldiers' feelings of deprivation did not correspond with objective conditions. Relative deprivation was theorized to account for high-ranking soldiers expressing more dissatisfaction than their lower-ranked counterparts, despite presumably better absolute living conditions. Furthermore, soldiers in units where promotion occurred frequently were less satisfied that those in units where promotion was rare. They found that higher-ranking officers were comparing themselves to those outside the military, or to other reference groups. Differences in individual frames of reference were found to be related to feelings of discontent and dissatisfaction i.e., the more people were promoted, the easier it is to be aware of others who are better off than oneself (Folger 1987). Thus, subjective dissatisfaction may not be a simple correlation with objective conditions, but derived through a comparative process with reference to others. Inherent in these comparisons are ideas of social justice such as fairness and equity, which serve to help individuals evaluate their outcomes.

Relative deprivation as a concept gained popularity after World War II, in part because of its inherent relationship to reference groups, which was then a topic of great interest within the field of sociology and psychology. Merton and Rossi's influential paper on identity helped to popularize the concept, leading to a long and varied history of investigation (Merton and Rossi 1957). Over the years, the concept of relative deprivation has acquired several meanings. Numerous models and specifications of the theory have been put forth, each focusing on different antecedents, intermediate factors, and consequences of feeling deprived. In addition, relative deprivation has been examined within various disciplines including sociology, social justice, social psychology, and economics—all of which differ somewhat in focus and methodology.

In discussing responses to social inequality in England, Runciman (1966) distinguished between two types of relative deprivation: egoistical, defined as feeling deprived in relation to others in one's group, and fraternal, identified as feelings of deprivation deriving from one's group being disadvantaged relative to another group. Crosby theorized that relative deprivation

14

required preconditions to be present such as perceived feasibility to obtain the outcome, entitlement to the outcome, lack of personal responsibility in attaining the outcome, and an available comparison possessing the outcome (Crosby 1976). In a subsequent study of discontent among working women, Crosby (1982) argued that entitlement is the essential antecedent to feeling relatively deprived when an outcome is desired. Folger (1987) attempts to overlay a theoretical framework called referent cognitions theory to further specify antecedents for relative deprivation. By including the psychological process of considering "what might have been" or the story one tells oneself about the evaluation of outcomes, Folger suggests that multiple scenarios of "what has been received compared to what was not, but might have been" can be mentally constructed with which to frame the evaluation of an outcome. According to Folger, discontent derives from the discrepancies of multiple comparisons between the actual outcomes and the awareness of a more favorable outcome (Folger 1987).

Although Crosby (1982) indicated that much of the empirical investigation has generally corroborated the expected associations between hypothesized antecedents and outcomes, critics have questioned the validity of relative deprivation on methodological grounds. Many of the studies were correlational, thereby preventing an adequate examination of causal links. In addition, relative deprivation has often been proffered as an explanation in a post-hoc fashion, precluding the necessary theoretical a priori specification of its determinants (Folger 1987). Relative deprivation has been used to explain several situations in which there are discrepancies between an individual's objective conditions and their subjective reactions to those experiences. For example, Strumpel (1976) found that objective measures of socioeconomic status were not significantly related to an individual's feelings of economic well-being. Research does not reveal that decreasing income influences financial dissatisfaction or living standards (Myers 1992). Similarly, experiences with the judicial system have not been found to correlate with level of dissatisfaction (Lind et al. 1990). Negative consequences such as incarceration or incurring litigation penalties do not significantly predict dissatisfaction with the experience. Relative deprivation has been defined to be comparative in nature, and to include how people feel about particular comparisons (Tyler et al. 1997). By definition, its comparative aspect, rather than its consequential subjective feelings, is what sets it apart from other models of cognitive judgments. Fundamental to this definition is the choice of what is termed the "comparison referent" or the comparison standard, the individual or group to which the comparison is being made. Studies indicate that people choose different reference standards in different situations (Merton and Rossi 1957). Research has found comparison standards to reflect both inferior and superior status positions relative to the index individual. Members of oppressed groups have been found to compare themselves with other individuals within disadvantaged groups, serving to establish a sense of group pride, reduce discontent, or maintain the social order (Major and Testa 1988). Specifically, some have advanced the concept of "relative advantage" to describe a comparison process in which individuals compared themselves with those of lower or inferior status (Wolf 1990).

Another aspect of the comparison standard is the level at which the comparison takes place. One may compare oneself as an individual or as a representative group member. Comparisons can be made to those similar to the self, or to refer back to themselves at other points in time. Similarly, group comparisons must include a choice of which group membership is to be chosen for the group comparison. Some suggest that context influences the choice of the comparison standard, or that people exhibit preferences for the specific types of comparisons (Oakes, Haslam, and Turner 1994). However, the weakness of a reference group theory such as relative deprivation lies in its inability to denote how reference groups or individuals are chosen for comparison (Buunk, Gibbons, and Reis-Bergan 1997). As a result, it is difficult to hypothesize which circumstance will determine whether one selects a superior or an inferior reference standard (Mirowsky 1987). Thus, social comparison processes may serve to either instill feelings of well-being and satisfaction, or to foster feelings of inadequacy and low self-esteem. Depending on the comparison standards, one could feel advantaged or deprived. Wilkinson's theory of relative deprivation within the public health arena suggests that those who live within a less egalitarian area, as evidenced by its level of income inequality, should experience increased morbidity and mortality relative to those within a more egalitarian area, regardless of absolute income level. While relative deprivation theory indicates that subjective satisfaction is not a simple response to objective outcomes (Tyler et al. 1997), but rather the result of social comparisons, it is possible to conceive that one might be relatively deprived in terms of material resources without perceiving themselves to be relatively deprived. For example, not having access to a computer to obtain relevant health information may render one relatively resource deprived without "feeling" deprived. It may be argued that not having access to a computer deprives one of fully participating in daily life within a particular society, given

16

the widespread use of technology in numerous spheres of everyday living. However, since Wilkinson does not specify this possibility within his hypotheses.

While empirical evidence suggests that reference standards may be of either inferior or superior position to the individual, Wilkinson does not address the issue that social comparisons may operate to establish and maintain financial satisfaction. If those within an area of widening income disparities compared themselves to those below them, this comparison may serve to bolster their perceptions of security and well-being, regardless of socioeconomic status. Due to the varying nature of comparison referents and the inability to accurately predict the choice of comparison referents, it remains unclear whether perceptions of deprivation relative to some perceived standard varies across and within different income levels to affect health outcomes.

Materialist Perspectives: Fundamental Cause

Theorists who embrace materialist perspectives give primacy to the absolute material conditions under which people live, even within the industrialized world. In contrast to psychosocial perspectives, these perspectives stress the role of material factors in influencing the SES-health association throughout the hierarchy. House and his colleagues began a line of research seeking to show how social stratification shapes health throughout the life course. House asserted that SES patterns the association between age and health by determining the exposure to, and impact of, social and biological mechanisms related to disease and death, with its greatest impact during middle and early old age (House et al. 1990). At lower socioeconomic levels, living conditions may influence the type and frequency of experiences thought to determine health and longevity (House et al. 1992).

Link and Phelan's Fundamental Cause (1995) hypothesis echoes these ideas, and further specifies how structural and material factors explain persisting health inequalities. They suggest that SES determines the distribution of resources, in the form of knowledge, money, power and or prestige, which, in turn, individuals use at every level of the hierarchy to reduce health risks and gain a health advantage. While new health threats emerge, those at the top of the hierarchy will always be best advantaged to reduce their risk of health hazards or mobilize themselves to employ health-protective strategies, regardless of the type of health challenge at any given time. In effect, this process serves to maintain the SES-health gradient. As such, Fundamental Cause seeks to explain the persistence of the SES-health association, particularly in the context of the developed world and despite increasing life expectancy.

This process of leveraging resources to gain an advantage is proposed to operate across multiple domains such as educational attainment, occupational status, location and quality of residence, etc., --all of which contribute to better health and longer life. Most importantly, this process is extremely dynamic, changing as new information about how to stay healthy, or prevent disease onset, becomes available. As a result, disease and death profiles change to reflect the social conditions and experiences under which we live, and will live in the future. Those conditions and experiences, however, are further patterned according to socioeconomic status.

Embedded within the Fundamental Cause explanation is the process of change—changes in social conditions over time, changes in diseases, responses to health threats, and changes in therapeutic and preventive technologies. Thus, this dynamic process of leveraging resources to reduce one's risk of disease and death is best exemplified from a historical perspective. In 1854, cholera killed 600 people within a quarter of a mile in the course of a few days in the Soho neighborhood of London. Until a local doctor, John Snow, demonstrated the link between cholera and a polluted public drinking pump, cholera was thought to spread through "miasma in the atmosphere" or divine intervention (Summers 1989). Families, rich and poor, were affected by this epidemic. Though once knowledge of the relationship between unsanitary water and cholera was confirmed, those at the top of the hierarchy were best positioned to use their resources to reduce their exposure to contaminated water, thereby reducing their risk of disease onset.

Today, most individuals within industrialized societies do not perish from infectious disease. Advances in the fields of bacteriology and virology have made many infectious diseases a scourge of the past, allowing chronic disease to emerge as the current challenge to health and longevity. However, our most recent infectious disease epidemic, HIV/AIDS, reveals a similar evolution to that of cholera in its relation to socioeconomic status. During its initial period of outbreak, HIV/AIDS struck both rich and poor alike. Until the routes of transmission were identified, and their respective risk reduction strategies employed, HIV/AIDS did not discriminate by social class. Although white gay men and intravenous drug users had initially comprised the largest segment of the infected population, education and income level did not

18

influence incidence or prevalence rates of the disease. However, once information related to risk-reduction became available, those with more resources could employ them to either mediate the course and consequences of disease once infected, or reduce risks through preventive strategies. As a result, HIV/AIDS is now a disease of lower income groups (Katz et al. 1998). In recent descriptions of the social patterning of this epidemic, many refer to the "changing face of HIV/AIDS" to describe the high incidence and prevalence among communities of color and low-income groups.

Susser and his colleagues described this dynamic process between health and social factors by reminding us "societies materially shape the way in which diseases are to be experienced" (Susser, Watson, and Hopper 1985). House and his colleagues further characterize this shaping of disease and death patterns by SES as that of a powerful river, whose course may be altered, but not blocked—a new course will simply emerge (House et al. 1990). For example, Winkleby and colleagues found education level to be highly associated with six risk factors for disease such as knowledge about health, cigarette smoking, hypertension, serum cholesterol, body mass index, and height, suggesting that education may operate to protect health by facilitating the adoption of positive values and attitudes, effective coping strategies, and entry into a social context where positive behaviors are normalized (Winkleby, Fortmann, and Barrett 1990). Link and Phelan indicate that resources such as knowledge or level of educational attainment may be leveraged in a myriad of ways to effect health (Link and Phelan 1995). In addition, when buttressed by concomitant resources such as income and wealth, individuals act to further employ self-care strategies to reduce risk. Some suggest it may be these very acts of human agency targeted at reducing morbidity and mortality on an individual level that operate to firmly link SES and health outcomes at the population level (Link et al. 1998).

Limitations of Current Research

While an individual-level analysis of disease and death in relation to SES and health-related strategies spanning decades, and even centuries, might prove the most direct and compelling test of this dynamic process explained by the Fundamental Cause perspective, data of this nature is not available (Link et al. 1998). Link and his colleagues have sought to explore situations where technological innovations have changed our ability to detect disease, such as mammography and pap smears, as opportunities to identify the shaping process (Link et al.

19

1998). While several explanations of how SES serves to shape morbidity and mortality differentials from a Fundamental Cause perspective have been put forth (Link et al. 1998; Link and Phelan 2000; Link and Phelan 1995), direct tests of the theory have not been undertaken. Similarly, while much attention has focused on examining whether the contextual effect of income inequality, per se, affects morbidity and/or mortality, little, if any, empirical analysis of its proposed mechanisms such as Relative Deprivation has been conducted.

The Need for Additional Research

Fundamental Cause and Relative Deprivation pose interesting, and not completely contradictory, explanations for the complex relationship between SES and health outcomes. Link and Phelan have argued that psychosocial processes such as relative deprivation are likely to be a component of the SES-health relationship, though not the driving force. However, little direct empirical investigation has been carried out to either support or refute these claims. As a critical first step to examining the validity of these perspectives, this work uses an analytical approach that poses the question, "If these explanations were true, what empirical evidence would we expect to find?" Within this analytic framework, assumptions are made that each perspective is valid.

Figure 2.1 illustrates the conceptual model for the analyses. This model depicts both the direct relationship of SES on health outcomes, as well as the two theorized pathways, relative deprivation and resource utilization, that are proposed to underlie this robust association. To test the relative contribution of each perspective, this analysis examines to what extent relative deprivation, as compared to health-related resource utilization as a function of SES, explains the SES variation in health outcomes.

Specific Aims and Hypotheses

To fully examine the relative merit of these two theoretical explanations, the specific aims of the work are to:
1) Examine and characterize the relationship between SES and Relative Deprivation as proposed by Wilkinson (1987) using the Health and Retirement Study (HRS) dataset. To test for potential confounding, analyses will also demographic characteristics such as race/ethnicity, age,

and marital status. I hypothesize that decreasing socioeconomic status is associated with relative deprivation, and relative deprivation is associated with health outcomes.

2) Examine and characterize the relationships between SES, Relative Deprivation, and three outcome variables: a) Self-Reported Health Status; b) Having a Life-threatening Condition; and b) All-Cause Mortality. I hypothesize that Relative Deprivation significantly reduces the size of the direct SES effect on health outcome variables.

3) Develop and validate a new measure, the Health-Related Resource Index (HRRI), which will reflect the extent to which a respondent engages in behaviors that are thought to promote health and longevity. Since it is virtually impossible to include all the behaviors that might be regarded as health-related resources, selected behaviors will serve to represent a larger set of behaviors, which have been found to reduce the risk of disease onset or progression. Thus, the HRRI will be utilized as a proxy measure of health-related resource utilization, a component within the broader process of general resource utilization.

4) Examine and characterize the relationship between SES and health-related resource utilization as hypothesized by Link and Phelan (1995). The relationship between SES and health-related resource utilization will control for age, race/ethnicity, and marital status. I hypothesize that higher socioeconomic status will be associated with health-related resource utilization, and will not differ in terms of age, gender, race/ethnicity, and marital status.

5) Examine the relationships between SES, health-related resource utilization, and three health outcome variables: a) Self-Reported Health Status; b) Having a Life-threatening Condition; and c) All-Cause Mortality. I hypothesize that higher SES will be directly associated with health-related resource utilization, and thereby, improve health status, reduce the likelihood of having a life-threatening condition, and increase survival. I also hypothesize that health-related resource utilization would decrease the size of the direct effect of SES on the outcome variables.

21

Figure 2.1: Conceptual Model

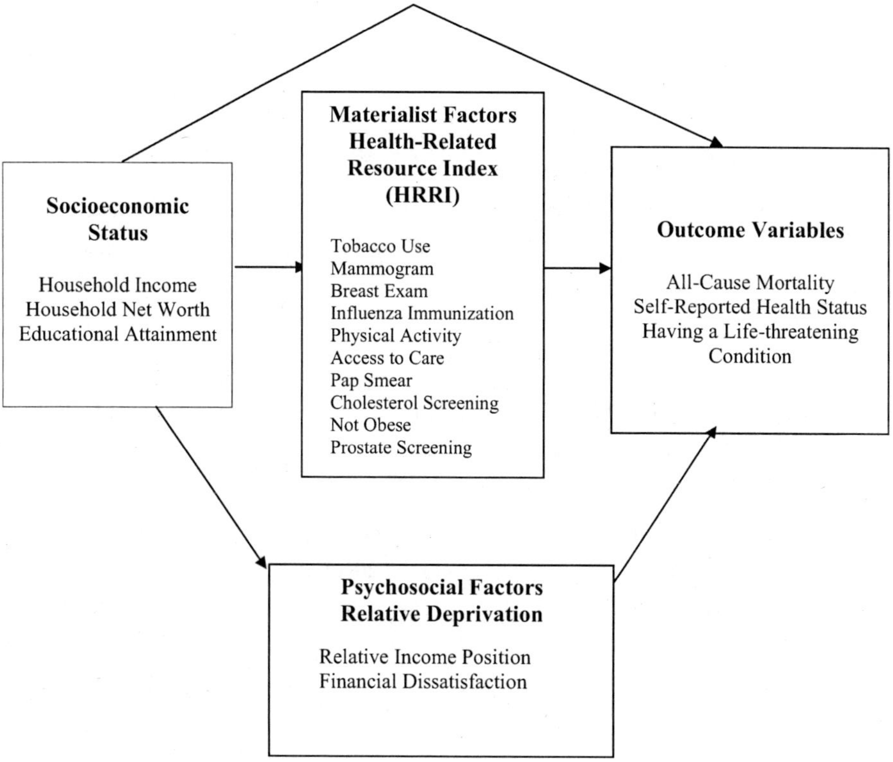

Socioeconomic Status

Household Income
Household Net Worth
Educational Attainment

Materialist Factors Health-Related Resource Index (HRRI)

Tobacco Use
Mammogram
Breast Exam
Influenza Immunization
Physical Activity
Access to Care
Pap Smear
Cholesterol Screening
Not Obese
Prostate Screening

Outcome Variables

All-Cause Mortality
Self-Reported Health Status
Having a Life-threatening Condition

Psychosocial Factors Relative Deprivation

Relative Income Position
Financial Dissatisfaction

Potential Confounders: Demographic Characteristics
Age
Race/Ethnicity
Marital Status

22

Chapter III

The Sample

The Dataset

The Health and Retirement Study (HRS), a nationally representative longitudinal data collection conducted by the University of Michigan Institute of Social Research and funded by the National Institute of Aging (NIA), is designed to examine the economic and social factors associated with retirement, health status, and quality of life in early old age. The HRS was launched in 1992 and sampled respondents aged 51-61 years old. The baseline interview was conducted in-person, and follow-up interviews are conducted by telephone every second year, with proxy interviews after death. Wave 1 of the HRS survey study began with an initial sample of over 12,600 persons in 7,600 households. Five waves of data collection have been completed to date.

The target population of the HRS survey includes all adults in the United States, born during the years 1931-1941. The observational unit, an eligible household, included at least one member who was aged 51-61 years old in 1992: 1) a single unmarried age-appropriate person; 2) a married couple in which both persons are age- appropriate; or 3) a married couple in which only one spouse is age- appropriate. Generally, the HRS has somewhat more women than men, resulting from the fact that in households where the age-eligible person is unmarried, that person is more likely to be a woman than a man. Persons living in institutions (nursing homes, long-term medical care or dependent care facilities, criminal justice facilities) were excluded from the HRS study.

HRS data includes a relatively unique composition of health and demographic information, as well as a comprehensive set of financial asset and liability indicators. As such, this data set is particularly appropriate for this study given its focus on the influence of economic factors with regard to disparities in health and longevity. Moreover, the age distribution of the sample is suitable since socioeconomic differences in health and longevity have been found to be greater in middle and early old age (House et al. 1990).

23

Sampling Design

The HRS sampling design is a multistage area probability sample of US households augmented by oversampling three subpopulations: African-Americans, Hispanics, and Floridians. Oversamples of African-Americans (1.86:1), Hispanics (1.72:1), and residents of the state of Florida (2:1) were obtained to increase the numbers of Black, Hispanic and Floridian respondents in order to conduct independent analysis within these subgroups. The sample included four stages of selection involving subsampling at successively smaller geographic areas. The primary stage of sampling involved probability proportionate to size (PPS) selection of U.S. Metropolitan Statistical Areas (MSAs) and non-MSA counties. A second stage included sampling of area segments (SSUs), comprised of Census block groups within sampled primary stage units (PSUs). Thirdly, all housing units (HUs) that were physically located within each of the selected SSU were enumerated, and a systematic selection of housing units from the HU listings for the sample SSUs was conducted. Lastly, an age-eligible person within a sample HU was selected. In order to match sample demographic distributions with known 1990 Census totals, post-stratification adjustments were made at both the household and person level.

Response Rates and Attrition

An important issue for all household surveys is the assessment of nonresponse bias. Response rates were calculated at both the household-level and the corresponding person-level for the HRS. All sample components attained or exceed the overall baseline response rate of 81.7 percent except the Hispanic supplement, which has a household response rate of 71 percent and a person-level response rate of 77 percent. Reinterview rates for 1994 and 1996 were respectively 91.8 percent and 93.1 percent. Estimates for the 1998 reinterview response rate is currently 93.8 percent, and estimates for 2000 have not been released to date.

Mortality rates for the original HRS respondents are approximately 2 percent between each wave, with the rates increasing from 1.8 percent between Waves 1 and 2, to 2.2 percent between 2 and 3, and 2.3 percent between Waves 3 and 4 (incomplete data). Participation patterns across the first four waves of data collection (1992, 1994, 1996, and 1998) indicate that 80.4 percent of the 12,523 baseline respondents have participated in all waves at which they were eligible, including those who have died. Of the remaining respondents, approximately 10

24

percent are missing one of the three follow-up interviews, close to 6 percent are missing two, and 4 percent have not participated in any of the follow up interviews.

Sample Weights

      The complex sample design of the HRS survey, which includes oversamples of Hispanic, Black, and Floridian households, requires weighting in analyses of the survey data. Sampling weights are used for each wave of data to compensate for the different probabilities of being selected into the sample as reflected in the various sampling rates of these subgroups. In addition, sample weights are used to reduce non-response bias, particularly in relation to geographic and race group differences. To ensure that the sample represents the target population, post-stratification adjustments at both the household and person level were developed by the HRS for each data collection year to match the sample demographic distributions of the March Current Population Surveys conducted by the US Census.

      The person-level weight integrates the household analysis weight with two other factors, the respondent selection weight and a post-stratification factor. The respondent selection weight is calculated as the inverse of the probability of selection of the age-appropriate respondent from the total number of age- appropriate household members. Data is also post-stratified to 1990 Census household totals by race and marital status, in addition to person-level adjustment by race/ethnicity, sex, and age to the 1990 PUMS estimates. Although the HRS did interview age-ineligible spouses or partners of age-appropriate respondents (51-61 years old), a person-level analysis should only include those representative of the population under investigation. Thus, non-zero person-level weights were given only to age-appropriate respondents, whereas age-ineligible respondents have a person-level weight of zero. For this study, base-year respondent weights (1992 and 1996) are used to model future events of the base-year population while adjusting for multistage sampling processes and oversampling.

      Standard dimensions for assessing data quality within surveys are sample size and response rate. Since the size of the standard errors depends on the sample size, sample size is a critical element of survey research. Response rate is an indicator of potential bias in that high rates of non-response are generally considered to render the sample non-representative of the population from which the sample was drawn, thus limiting the validity of making valid inferences. Given the sample size (smallest cohort =2,705) and the response rate of the HRS, this data set can be considered an adequate sample from which to test the hypothesized relationships.

Missing Data

Missing data often represents a major problem in survey measurement of financial variables, especially the measurement of household wealth (Juster and Suzman 1995). In many instances, conventional imputation procedures assign a value to the missing component, assuming that the distribution of missing values is approximately the same as known data values for respondents with similar demographic characteristics. To reduce the level of missing data for economic variables that are generally subject to high rates of non-response, the Health and Retirement Study utilized a method that included a series of questions referring to a "bracket" rather than an exact "amount" when respondents could or would not provide a precise estimate of financial information. A bracket question specifies a rounded dollar amount from which the respondent is asked to estimate whether a financial component is more or less than the specified amount. This unfolding technique allowed responses to be categorized using an estimated value supplied by the respondent. HRS analysts used the responses to the "bracket" questions to produce missing value imputation for total household income and total household net worth using the SAS program, IMPUTE (Cao 2001). This unfolding bracket method is thought to have significantly improved the quality of economic data by imputing reasonable values for those that were missing (Wilson 2001; Hill 1999).

The study sample for the relative deprivation analyses includes respondents from Wave 1 who also have outcome measurements at Wave 4. Wave 1 is selected to mark the beginning of the observation period since the dissatisfaction items were only included in Wave1. The study sample for the resource utilization analyses includes respondents from Wave 3 who also have outcome measurements at Wave 4. Wave 3 is selected to mark the beginning of this observation period since the preventive health behavior items used to construct the Health-related Resource Index were not included in Waves 1 and 2. Hence, it is necessary to exclude Waves 1 and 2 from the resource utilization analyses. However, selecting these different observation periods does not threaten the validity of the analyses since the purpose of the study is not to directly compare the cohorts, but rather to test each theoretical framework using its respective cohort.

Data were not available for each study variable for all respondents in the HRS Wave1, Wave 3 or Wave 4 samples. While it is generally not recommended to exclude individuals with missing information, Korn and Graubaud (1999) suggest dropping observations when a small amount of item nonresponse exists. In addition, values for zip code, county or state of residence could not be imputed. Thus, for the relative deprivation sample, observations were dropped for: 1) those respondents with missing values for Wave 1 and Wave 4 self-reported health status (.01%); 2) those respondents with missing values for zip code, county or state of residence (1.9%); and 3) those respondents who had "missing" for race/ethnicity (.2%). Values were imputed for missing dissatisfaction items by calculating the mean of non-missing dissatisfaction items by gender, and substituting the gender-specific mean for each missing value. Case deletion and imputations procedures resulted in a final sample of 9,992 respondents for HRS Wave 1/4 (a 2.2% reduction of the total sample of those in both Waves 1 and 4). Financial dissatisfaction, however, is not imputed in analyses where it serves as the dependent variable.

For the resource utilization analysis, observations were dropped for: 1) those respondents who reported "missing organ" for the prostate, cervix, or breast (.2%); 2) those female respondents who had 6 or more missing values out of a possible total of 9 health-related resource items such as mammogram, health insurance, and body weight, and male respondents who had 4 or more missing values out of a possible total of 7 health-related resource items such as physically active and prostate screening (.05%); 3) those respondents with missing values for Wave 4 self-reported health status (.05%); (4) those respondents who had "missing" for any of the other demographic study variables including marital status (.02%), race/ethnicity (.2%), and age (.1%); and 5) those respondents with missing values for SES variables including educational attainment, household income and household net worth (.1%). Values were imputed for missing health-related resource items by calculating the respondent's mean of non-missing resource items, and imputing their mean for each missing value. Case deletion and imputation procedures resulted in a final sample of 9,884 respondents for HRS Wave 3/4 (a 1.1% reduction of the total sample of those in both Waves 3 and 4). The following table indicates the types of analysis, the base and termination year, and study sample size for the various analyses.

Table 3.1. Analytic Study Sample Description

Relative Deprivation Analyses							
Type of Analysis	Baseline Wave	Termination Wave	Total Sample Size	Study Sample Size	% Reduction	% Mortality (n)	Study Cohort Size
Prospective	Wave 1 (1992)	Wave 4 (1998)	10,218	9,992	2.2%	6.2% (769)	8,012
Resource Utilization Analyses							
Type of Analysis	Baseline Wave	Termination Wave	Total Sample Size	Study Sample Size	% Reduction	% Mortality	Study Cohort Size
Prospective	Wave 3 (1996)	Wave 4 (1998)	9,990	9,884	1.1%	2.5% (267)	7,774

Constructing the Analytic Sample

HRS data is available in two versions, an unrestricted public-use file and a restricted-use file. The public-use files including data, codebook and user files were downloaded from the HRS website (http://www.umich.edu/~hrswww/). To eliminate the possibility (though presumably small) of a transfer, extraction, or a conversion problem when receiving data, particularly in relation to downloading files from the Internet, all variables and records within each data file were checked against data documentation information. All variables used in the analyses were also examined for inconsistencies and outliers.

The HRS restricted data includes highly sensitive identifying information such as respondents' location of residence and occupation. To ensure confidentiality, the University of Michigan required the restricted data be obtained through a contractual agreement specifying stringent data protection procedures and Columbia University IRB approval (CPMC IRB approval #14122, 1/2/02). Obtaining respondent residential location from the HRS restricted data file enables one to link 1990 Census estimates of median household income at each of the geographical aggregations to each respondent, an essential component for this study. Median household income estimates for each zip code, county, and state were extracted from the 1990 US Census data files using CensusCD1990+Maps (GeoLytics 1997), a software package available at the Columbia University Electronic Data Service (EDS). The HRS restricted data and the 1990 Census data were merged with the HRS public use files for those analyses examining relative income.

28

All analyses within this study were stratified by gender. This procedure is adopted for several reasons. First, gender-specific preventive health behavior items such as mammograms could not be included within a generic index of resource utilization. As a result, gender-specific indexes were developed and thus, required separate analyses. Secondly, survey data are greatly influenced by illness and prevention orientations, health reporting behavior and physical status--- all of which are thought to explain sex differentials in morbidity and mortality (Verbrugge and Wingard 1987). Thirdly, behavioral patterns differ by gender and age (Liang et al. 1999). Lastly, gender significantly influences the economic orientation and status of individuals. In an effort to reduce the influence of these social factors, analyses were conducted separately for males and females.

To examine the mediating processes of relative deprivation and resource utilization on health outcomes over time, cohorts were constructed to reflect those with favorable health at baseline. For the relative deprivation analyses, a female and male cohort limited to those who reported good/very good/excellent health at baseline (w1) is used to assess the likelihood of a decline in self-rated health status to fair/poor at w4. In addition, a female and male cohort limited to those respondents who reported no life-threatening conditions at w1 is used to examine the likelihood of developing any life-threatening conditions at w4. Similarly, female and male cohorts of those with good/excellent health and without any life-threatening conditions at w3 were used to examine the likelihood of a decline in health status to fair/poor and developing any life-threatening condition at w4 for the resource utilization analyses.

Gender-specific prospective cohorts were also constructed to examine the likelihood of dying during the two observation periods (w1-- w4, and w3-- w4). To determine the likelihood of death in relation to relative deprivation, male and female cohorts included respondents who participated in wave 1 and were reinterviewed at wave 4. Likewise, male and female respondents who participated in wave 3 are included to determine the role of resource utilization as it relates to SES and mortality at wave 4.

Chapter IV

Methods and Measurement of Variables

Statistical Methods

This study utilizes both bivariate and multivariable statistical methods to provide empirical support for the hypothesized relationships. First, crosstabs and correlations are conducted between each independent variable and each dependent variable to determine the nature of relationships between all variables. Secondly, two types of multivariable methods are employed: logistic and linear regression. Logistic regression is employed for those analyses that examine dichotomous outcomes, and linear regression is used for outcomes measured continuously.

Stata, version 6.0, an integrated statistical software package for research professionals, is used for all data management and statistical procedures (StataCorp 1999). Complex survey designs such as the HRS employ sampling strategies including stratification, clustering, and differential selection probabilities. Because of the sampling design, observations within the same cluster are not independent. Since most software packages estimate standard errors under the assumption of simple random sampling and independence of observations, one needs to employ sampling adjustments to correct for the underestimation of variances. To obtain appropriate variance estimates, a Taylor Series linearization method available in Stata is employed in all analyses. Specifically, the Stata program allows the specification of HRS survey design information such as sampling weights, strata and primary sampling unit variables to calculate point estimates of population parameters and correct standard errors, p-values, and confidence intervals for those estimates.

Rationale for Prospective Design

Panel designs, such as the HRS, are repeated observations on the same sample of individuals over time (Finkel 1995). Analyzing outcomes over time on the same sample of individual cases often provides stronger causal evidence because it explicitly includes the temporal ordering of events, an essential condition of causal inference (Menard 1991). Drawing on this distinctive feature of the HRS, a classic epidemiological prospective design is employed by constructing several cohorts of respondents who reported either good/excellent health or did not have any life-threatening condition, and following them over time to track the onset of either

30

poor health or a life-threatening condition. The prospective cohort design compares each subject to him or herself, which facilitates the study of hypothesized processes in relation to health outcomes over time.

Causal models often assume that the relationship between X and Y occurs in one direction i.e. X influences Y, but not the opposite (Finkel 1995). If the temporal ordering sequence between variables is clear, this assumption may be appropriate. However, the causal sequence of variables is not always understood. This is made abundantly clear when examining the role of health-related resource utilization in relation to health outcomes. Initial findings indicated that the higher the level of employing risk-reduction behaviors such as mammograms and cholesterol screening, the more likely a respondent is to have a life-threatening condition. This counterintuitive finding suggested the possibility of a non-recursive relationship in that having any life-threatening conditions may influence one's engagement in preventive health behaviors as a result of being under a provider's care. The prospective cohort design enables one to separate out the process of utilizing health-related resources from engaging in behaviors as a result of being in the care system by restricting the cohort to those who report no life-threatening conditions at baseline.

Measuring Socioeconomic Status

Social scientists have used the term "socioeconomic status" to represent the relative position of an individual within a social hierarchy. Socioeconomic status is typically conceptualized from the vantage point of Weber's ideas of stratification including income, education, occupation, and ownership of property. Although several indicators are often used to measure SES, it is frequently discussed as a one-dimensional construct similar to other "status" measures, reflecting a static position within a categorical range of values. However, the different SES indicators measure distinct but related aspects of this complex concept (Rogers, Hummer, and Nam 2000; Duncan and Petersen 2001). While composite indices have been used in the past, it is now recommended that several indicators be used to differentiate the associations between the components embedded within the multidimensional nature of SES (Liberatos, Link, and Kelsey 1988; Williams and Collins 1995).

Some have suggested that education is the most stable, robust and convenient indicator (Liberatos, Link, and Kelsey 1988). Its ease of measurement, applicability to those not in the

31

labor force, and stability over time has made it one of the most widely used indicators of SES (Krieger, Williams, and Moss 1997). Although educational attainment is typically measured as years of school completed, completion of degrees such as high school or college can also provide critical information about accomplishments and skills. A high school diploma often translates into better employment opportunities, suggesting that certifications may be more important than years of schooling completed. Education has been found to directly influence health status and mortality through health behaviors, and indirectly through its effect on income production and occupational status (Elo and Preston 1996). However, education as a measure of SES does have its limitations. The relatively minor change in educational status in adulthood can preclude determining how health status is affected by change in educational attainment, and the benefits from educational attainment have been found to vary by race and gender (Williams and Collins 1995). Moreover, educational attainment varies by the age cohort of the individual and region of the country (Liberatos, Link, and Kelsey 1988). As such, educational attainment may incorrectly estimate the effects of SES if used as a single indicator.

Income level has also been found to be a strong predictor of morbidity and mortality, especially for persons under the age of 65 (Coburn and Pope 1974). Measures of income typically include respondent's income, income per capita, poverty rates or household income. As with education, each income measure has advantages and disadvantages. While respondent's income ignores other income sources within the household, household income often does not take into consideration the size of the family (Hummer, Rogers, and Eberstein 1998). Unfortunately, questions about income often result in high nonresponse, and tend to change over time more so than education or occupation (Duncan 1996).

Prior to the mid 1980s, wealth had been typically assessed in studies of the very rich, and largely ignored when examining stratification processes within the broader population (Spilerman 2000). Research largely focused on labor market earnings without regard to a family's command over material resources. However, as equity acquisition has increased across the spectrum of households in America and wealth data has been made increasingly available, many have recommended supplementing the estimation of SES by including indicators of wealth (Williams and Collins 1995; Conley 1999). Wealth accumulates over time, is less affected by income fluctuations, and provides a better overall measure of access to resources, particularly in people who are retired or are preparing to retire (Feinstein 1993; Land and Russel 1996). As a source of economic security, wealth reflects a household's ability to endure financial hardship such as unemployment or illness (Krieger, Williams, and Moss 1997), and thus, be of greater value in estimating the depth of economic resource capacity.

To comprehensively assess the unique and conjoint aspects of social position, three indicators are used for this study: total household income, total household wealth, and educational attainment. The total household income measure represents personal income items such as wage and salary from any job; bonuses, overtime, tips, and commission income; income from a professional practice or trade; other income from work, including second jobs or the military reserves; unemployment compensation; worker's compensation; veterans' benefits; retirement pensions; annuities; Supplemental Security Income; and Social Security income. In addition, other income sources are included such as income from private businesses, farms, professional practices or partnerships, rental income; dividend or interest income; trust fund or royalty income; alimony or child support; any financial support provided by friends or relatives; inheritances, gifts, or loans of any kind; and food stamps or welfare payments (Moon and Juster 1995).

Wealth is the net worth of a household, typically accumulated through inheritance, investment, and other forms of savings. The net worth measure is calculated by adding up the current value of all assets a household owns (bank accounts, stocks, bonds, life insurance savings, mutual fund shares, houses, unincorporated businesses, consumer durables such as cars and major appliances, and the value of pension rights), then subtracting the value of all liabilities (consumer debt, mortgage balances, and other outstanding debt). Essentially, non-housing equity is added to housing equity. Individual housing equity items in the wealth calculation includes ownership of home, farmland, mobile home, multiple dwelling, and the sum of all mortgages held on such property. Non-housing equity items include liquid assets such as cash, stock, mutual funds, investment trusts, and vehicles.

Household income is measured using the natural logs of the original household income values to reduce the skew of the income distribution (Osborne 2002). Household net worth is also modified using the natural log transformation, after the distribution is adjusted upwards and anchored at 1 to eliminate negative values. Although categorical milestones such as degree certification may be valuable in measuring accomplishments, educational attainment is measured

33

continuously as the highest grade of school or year of college completed (0-17 years, with 17 representing post-baccalaureate education) to include all available data.

Measuring Relative Deprivation

Although social comparison processes such as relative deprivation have been extensively explored within the disciplines of sociology, psychology, social justice, and economics, the conceptualization of the concept as it applies to health needs further development. Some studies have attempted to capture theorized antecedents of this construct by measuring the extent of income inequality, a contextual variable, at various geographic levels (Kennedy, Kawachi, and Prothrow-Stith 1996; Kawachi et al. 1997; Lynch et al. 1998). Although researchers postulate that within areas of increased income disparity, one is more likely to engage in social comparison processes, studies have not been conducted to examine this claim. Research has focused on demonstrating the effects of income inequality at various geographic aggregations, but not whether inequality leads to social comparison, nor how social comparison affects health outcomes.

Others have measured theorized consequences of relative deprivation such as shame, low self-esteem, low social capital, distrust, and reduced participation in civic activities (Wilkinson 1996; Kawachi et al. 1997) (Wilkinson 1999). While these studies demonstrate a higher incidence of these psychosocial factors within areas of higher inequality, it is not clear whether social comparison processes underpin this relationship.

According to Wilkinson's hypothesis, it matters more where you are in the social hierarchy relative to those around you, rather than one's absolute position along the spectrum, and individuals who feel relatively deprived experience low self-esteem and shame. For this research study, relative deprivation is operationalized using two measures: a constructed variable of relative income difference and financial dissatisfaction. Relative income difference is a continuous measure calculated as the difference between the respondent's logged household income and the log of the median household income of the respondent's respective state, county and zip code. Although it's unclear how to define an appropriate reference group, some evidence suggests that the level of geographic aggregation influences the pathways through which contextual factors may be translated into individual risk (Soobader and LeClere 1999). Thus, measures of relative income are calculated at three different geographic aggregations: zip code, county and state. The median household income within these areas is selected to approximate a community income norm. The purpose of the relative income difference score is to directly measure a respondent's income position or "rank" in relation to a geographically defined estimate of community income.

Dissatisfaction with one's financial situation is examined as a potential indicator of relative deprivation. Preliminary analyses of this indicator suggested that it might be related to relative deprivation in that people can feel dissatisfied with their financial situation, regardless of income level. Contrary to income or assets which are material goods, financial dissatisfaction is similar to relative deprivation in that it is a psychosocial construct. As such, financial dissatisfaction may be considered to be a component of the hierarchical stress that according to Wilkinson derives from feeling relatively deprived. One could assume that if one feels relatively deprived, they should also be dissatisfied with their financial situation. The financial dissatisfaction indicator reflects the response to the question, "How satisfied or dissatisfied are you with your own financial situation at the current time? Financial dissatisfaction is categorically coded as follows: 1=very satisfied, 2=somewhat satisfied, 3=evenly satisfied, 4=somewhat dissatisfied and 5=very dissatisfied.

To discern whether financial dissatisfaction is a function of being generally dissatisfied rather than reflecting a dissatisfaction with one's financial situation, two additional indicators are included: dissatisfaction with life in general and interpersonal dissatisfaction. These dissatisfaction indicators represent domains considered to be unrelated to financial issues. Dissatisfaction with life represents a global measure of one's general dissatisfaction indicated by the response to a single question, "How satisfied or dissatisfied are you with your life as a whole? Life dissatisfaction is coded into five categories with 1 representing "very satisfied" and 5 representing "very unsatisfied." Interpersonal dissatisfaction is measured by an index calculated as the sum of the answers to four questions about how satisfied the respondent is with their friendships, family life, handling problems in general, and their neighborhood. Responses to individual dissatisfaction questions range from 1 (very satisfied) to 5 (very dissatisfied) which sum to a possible score of 4 to 20 for interpersonal dissatisfaction.

Measuring Health-related Resource Utilization

Fundamental Cause theory focuses on access to and utilization of resources, a process which reflects an individual's knowledge of and access to health-protective and risk reduction strategies to confer a health advantage (Link and Phelan 1995). For example, the process of employing technological innovations such as cancer detection screens has been shown to be significantly related to education and income (Link et al. 1998). For those who function at higher cognitive levels, educational resources may be easily applied to the ever-changing health information to promote one's health (Kenkel 1991). Similarly, engaging in health-promoting behaviors such as physical activity may be indicative of using health-related knowledge to improve health and longevity.

Although the Fundamental Cause hypothesis has been elucidated in several articles (Link and Phelan 1995; Link and Phelan 1995; Link and Phelan 1996; Link and Phelan 2000), resource utilization has not been operationalized and tested as a causal mechanism. While Link and colleagues present an example of the distribution of mammography and pap smears by educational attainment as reflective of SES shaping the employment of health-related technologies (Link et al. 1998), utilization of health-related technology has not been examined in relation to health outcomes.

If one assumes that individuals leverage their educational and financial resources to employ health-promoting strategies, one would expect that resource-rich individuals should employ health-related technological innovations and healthy lifestyle behaviors, reflecting both a knowledge and understanding of health information as well as financial resources to employ these strategies. While many behaviors related to health promotion have been shown to be patterned by SES (Novotny et al. 1988; Ford et al. 1991; Ford et al. 1994; Eisen et al. 1999), empirical evidence indicates that healthy lifestyle behaviors alone do not significantly explain the association between SES and health outcomes (Lantz et al. 1998). However, Link and Phelan contend that health-related resource utilization includes a vast array of health-relevant entities such as problem-solving abilities, occupational conditions, social relationships, and environmental exposures (Link and Phelan 2000).

Drawing on the work of Link and colleagues, a Health-Related Resource Index, the HRRI, is constructed to measure this construct. The HRRI reflects the extent to which an individual engages in both healthy lifestyle behaviors and employs preventive health behavior technologies such as mammography and prostate screening. Access to care is also included in the index as a resource related to the context in which an individual works. Ideally, one would include a myriad of factors from different domains that are considered to improve health and well-being. The purpose of this indicator is not to measure the extent of engaging in these specific behaviors per se, but rather to use this index as a proxy to represent the extent to which one employs the larger universe of health-related resources. The HRRI items are selected to represent strategies that necessitate using one's knowledge of health promotion and disease prevention, as well as the resources to access them.

Preliminary analyses of the relationship between the percentage of respondents who employed one health-related resource, and the percentage of respondents who employed the remainder of the selected health-related resources indicated that the possibility of exposure to any one health behavior increases the likelihood of engaging in the remaining health behaviors, suggesting that individuals with resources such as knowledge, money, power, prestige, and social connections tend to engage in an array of behaviors reflecting a tendency for utilizing resources to protect one's health

This new measure, the Health-related Resource Index, is a gender-specific index that includes some of the leading health indicators chosen for Healthy People 2010 (U.S. Department of Health and Human Services 2000). Gender-specific indexes are constructed to reflect the exclusive items for males and females. For example, the HRRI for males includes prostate screening while the female HRRI includes mammography. To enable one to compare and contrast resource utilization models to the relative deprivation analyses, all models are analyzed separately by gender. The indicators that comprise the female HRRI are: 1) Non-smoking status, 2) Not Obese, 3) Physically Active, 4) Mammogram, 5) Access to Health Care, 6) Breast Exam, 7) Pap Smear, 8) Influenza Immunization, and 9) Cholesterol Screening. For males, the index includes 1) Non-smoking status, 2) Not Obese, 3) Physically Active, 4) Access to Health Care, 5) Influenza Immunization, 6) Cholesterol Screening and 7) Prostate Screening. Non-smoking status is measured as never having smoked cigarettes. Not Obese is coded as those respondents having a body mass index (BMI) score of less than 30 and more than 18.5. BMI is calculated as [Weight in pounds ÷ Height in inches ÷ Height in inches] x 703 (Centers for Disease Control 2002). Physically active is represented as those respondents reporting participation in vigorous physical activity or exercise such as sports, heavy housework, or a job that involves physical

37

labor three times a week or more. Access to health care is measured as having any type of public or private health insurance.

While access to care, measured as having health insurance, may play a role in an individual's engagement in some of the screening procedures, and thus be causally related, studies have also found that SES disparities in preventive care persist regardless of health insurance status (Katz and Hofer 1994). Moreover, health insurance is not causally related to the other health behavior items such as smoking, body mass and physical activity. Thus, access to care is included in the index rather than being used as a control variable.

As a new measure of the health-resource utilization process, the individual health-related resources items are analyzed as separate variables as well as examined as an index to explore the utility of the HRRI. Each resource item is dichotomized (yes=1; no=0), and summed to create a score reflecting the extent of health-related resource utilization for females and males, respectively.

Measuring Health Outcomes

The dependent variables, self-reported health status, having any life-threatening conditions, and all-cause mortality, have been used in numerous landmark studies to assess health outcomes (House et al. 1994; Ross and Wu 1995). Self-rated health has been found to be a valid and reliable measure of general physical well being, and is highly correlated with other "objective" measures such as physician assessments (Idler and Benyamini 1997). The self-rated overall health status item in the HRS is derived from the National Health Interview Survey (NHIS). Self-rated health is the respondent's subjective assessment of his or her general health (1=excellent, 2=very good, 3=good, 4=fair, 5=poor), which is collapsed into a 2-category variable for analysis: 0=excellent/very good/ good, and 1=fair/poor.

Assessing the onset of conditions is thought to capture the recent health experiences of respondents and may indicate possible pathways to health after middle age (Hayward et al. 2000). Moreover, it is also considered to be a less subjective health outcome as compared to self-reported health status (Ross and Mirowsky 2000). However, this measure reflects responses to whether a doctor ever told a respondent they have a particular condition. As such, this self-report measure may contain bias in that it reflects, in part, access to and utilization of the health care system. Nonetheless, many of these conditions represent the leading causes of death in the

38

early retirement years (51-61 years old), indicating that the onset of serious conditions is firmly linked to health outcomes. Having any life-threatening conditions is calculated by summing dichotomously coded responses to five questions (Yes=1, and No=0): "Has a doctor ever told you that you have....1) diabetes, 2) cancer, 3) chronic lung disease, 4) heart disease, and 5) stroke. This calculation is then coded dichotomously as 1=having any life-threatening conditions and 0=having no life-threatening conditions.

All-Cause Mortality is coded dichotomously (dead=1; alive=0), reflecting death prior to the time of the follow-up interview. Death status is verified against the National Death Index for respondents who have died up until 1995. For those respondents who have died since 1995, death information reflects the report of interviewers from informant report.

Measuring Control Variables

Demographic characteristics such as race, age, and marital status are included as control variables. Since these variables are related to SES, health-related behaviors, and health status, they are included in the analyses as potential confounders. Race/ethnicity is the respondent's subjective assessment of his or her racial and ethnic origins. It is categorically coded in response to the questions, "Do you consider yourself primarily white or Caucasian, Black or African-American, American Indian, or Asian, or something else?" and "Do you consider yourself Hispanic or Latino? (1= White/Caucasian, 2=Black/African-American, 3=Hispanic/Latino 4=Other). Four dummy variables are then constructed from this categorical race/ethnicity variable, and Black/African-American is used as the referent category. Age is coded in years old at time of interview. Marital status is coded dichotomously as married (defined as married or living with a partner), and unmarried (defined as separated, widowed, divorced or never married).

Description of the Study Cohort

Table 4.1 presents a description of the cohort study variables under investigation for the relative deprivation analysis. Independent variables reflect baseline year information (1992), while dependent variables reflect termination year data (1998). Weighted and unweighted descriptors are included for all variables. In terms of the women, the mean age is approximately 60 years old; 86% are Caucasian, and two-thirds report being married or cohabitating (75%).

Educational attainment indicated the completion of some years of college education on average (12.7 years). With respect to health outcomes, 18% reported poor health status and 30% reported having a life-threatening condition.

For men, the average age is slightly younger at approximately 56 years old, and 89% of the men reported being married or cohabitating—almost a 15% difference as compared to the women. Educational attainment indicated that some college education is completed on average, though it's slightly higher as compared to the women (13.1 years). While fewer men report poor health status (16%) than women, they also report a slightly higher proportion of having a life-threatening condition (35%). As would be expected from national death trends, the proportion of mortality is higher for men (6.6%) than women (4.1%).

Table 4.2 presents a description of the cohort study variables under investigation for the resource utilization analysis. Both weighted and unweighted descriptors are included for all variables. Independent variables reflect baseline year information (1996), while dependent variables reflect termination year data (1998). As such, the participants for the resource utilization analysis are four years older than those in the relative deprivation cohort due to the difference in the baseline years. As expected, the mean age for the women is approximately 65 years old (64.7 years). The majority of the women are Caucasian (85%) and over two-thirds report being married or cohabitating (71%). Their mean level of years of education completed is 12.7 years. In terms of health outcomes, 12% report poor health status and over one-quarter (28%) report having a life-threatening condition.

The males under investigation for the resource utilization analysis reported an average age of approximately 65 (64.6), almost identical to the women in this cohort. Both average educational attainment (13.1 years) and proportion of those reporting being married or cohabitating among men (84%) are higher as compared to the women in this cohort. While men report a similar proportion of poor health status (13%) as compared to women, a higher proportion of having a life-threatening condition (34%) is reported for men.

Table 4.1 Distribution of Cohort Study Variables at W1,1992: Relative Utilization Analysis		
Females (N=4,378)		
Independent Variables	Unweighted	Weighted (s.d.)
Demographic Factors Mean Age	53.7	55.9 (.05)
Race/ethnicity Caucasian/White	77%	86%
African American/Black	14%	8%
Hispanic	7%	4%
Other	2%	2%
Marital Status Married/Cohabitating	82%	75%
Unmarried/Widowed/Divorced	18%	25%
Socioeconomic Status Mean Educational Attainment	12.5	12.7 (.08)
Mean Log Household Income	$1,056 (108)	$1,053
Mean Log Household Net Worth	$1,100 (296)	$1,119
Relative Deprivation Mean Log Zip Code Income Difference	$29 (104)	$20
Mean Financial Dissatisfaction	2.3	2.2 (.03)
Mean Interpersonal Dissatisfaction	6.0	5.9 (.05)
Mean Life Dissatisfaction	1.5	1.5 (.02)
Dependent Variables		
Health Outcomes at Wave 4 Poor Health Status	16%	18%
Having Any Life-threatening Conditions	29%	30%
Mortality	4.3%	4.1%
Males(N=3,634)		
Demographic Factors Mean Age	56.8	55.7(5.0)
Race/ethnicity Caucasian/White	80%	87%
African American/Black	11%	6%
Hispanic	7%	5%
Other	2%	2%
Marital Status Married/Cohabitating	92%	89%
Unmarried/Widowed/Divorced	8%	11%
Socioeconomic Status Mean Educational Attainment (s.d.)	12.7	13.1 (.09)
Mean Log Household Income (s.d.)	$1069 (104)	$1078
Mean Log Household Net Worth (s.d.)	$1119 (279)	$1125
Relative Deprivation Mean Log Zip Code Income Difference	$40 (99)	$43
Mean Financial Dissatisfaction	2.2	2.2 (.034)
Mean Interpersonal Dissatisfaction	5.6	5.7 (.08)
Mean Life Dissatisfaction	1.4	1.5 (.03)
Dependent Variables		
Health Outcomes at Wave 4 Poor Health Status	18%	16%
Having Any Life-threatening Conditions	37%	35%
Mortality	8.2%	6.6%

Table 4.2 Distribution of Cohort Study Variables at W3, 1996: Resource Utilization Analysis				
	Females (N=4,289)		Males (N=3,485)	
Independent Variables	Unweighted	Weighted (s.d.)	Unweighted	Weighted (s.d.)
Demographic Factors Mean Age	62.6	64.7 (.04)	65.8	64.6 (.06)
Race/ethnicity				
Caucasian/White	77%	85%	80%	85%
African American/Black	15%	9%	11%	8%
Hispanic	6%	4%	7%	5%
Other	2%	2%	2%	2%
Marital Status				
Married/Cohabitating	75%	71%	88%	84%
Unmarried/Widowed/Divorced	25%	29%	12%	16%
Socioeconomic Status Mean Household Income	$56,164	$54,656 (1,754)	$66,613	$74,684 (2,689)
Mean Household Net Worth	$230,227	$265,653 (14,721)	$272,139	$299,137 (16,731)
Resource Utilization Access to Health Care	79%	78%	86%	84%
Breast Exam	63%	62%		
Cholesterol Level Screening	69%	70%	69%	68%
Influenza Immunization	35%	38%	36%	34%
Mammogram	73%	74%		
Non-Smoking Status	78%	79%	77%	77%
Not Obese (BMI <30)	73%	76%	77%	77%
Pap Smear	71%	70%		
Physically Active	52%	53%	62%	62%
Prostate Screening			67%	66%
Mean Health-related Resource Index (HRRI)	5.9	6.0 (.05)	4.58	4.7 (.04)
Dependent Variables				
Health Outcomes at Wave 4 Poor Health Status	13%	12%	15%	13%
Having Any Life-threatening Conditions	27%	28%	36%	34%
Mortality	1.7%	1.7%	3.1%	2.5%

Chapter V

SES, Relative Deprivation, and Health Outcomes

This chapter tests Wilkinson's hypothesis that relative deprivation underlies the
association between socioeconomic status (SES) and health (Wilkinson 1997b). According to
Wilkinson, socioeconomic status is related to health within western societies not so much
because of absolute deprivation but because of relative deprivation. SES influences the extent to
which people feel deprived in comparison to others and this relative deprivation is related to
health. Figure 5.1 depicts Wilkinson's theory.

Figure 5.1 Relative Deprivation Causal Model

SES $\longrightarrow$ Relative $\longrightarrow$ Health Outcome

                  Deprivation

Recall that two indicators measure relative deprivation: relative income and financial
dissatisfaction. Relative income was calculated as the difference between a respondent's
household income and their respective median zip code income level to determine a rank
position within their community. Financial dissatisfaction was a self-reported assessment scale
of how satisfied one is with respect to their financial situation. This psychosocial measure of
financial dissatisfaction was included as an indicator of the consequence of feeling relatively
deprived as described by Wilkinson. If relative deprivation mediates the association between
SES and health, the SES-health relationship will be explained or accounted for by the measure of
relative deprivation. Results must also indicate that compared with those whose income is below
the median, those with incomes above their respective zip code median income level experience
better health outcomes. Specifically, relative deprivation should be directly related to health
outcomes such that adjustment for relative deprivation should significantly reduce the
association between SES and health. On the other hand, if controlling relative deprivation fails
to reduce the SES-health association or if relative deprivation is correlated to health when SES is
controlled, mediation cannot be inferred. Analyses are presented with reference to specific
questions that separate the possible associations between SES, relative deprivation, and health

43

outcomes so as to evaluate whether those associations support Wilkinson's hypothesis. The
analysis begins with the basic questions such as:

Is SES associated with health and longevity in the HRS dataset?

Figure 5.2   SES—Health Outcomes Model

SES ⟶ Health Outcome

Bivariate analyses are conducted to examine the relationship between SES indicators and
health outcomes. The sample was divided into five quintiles according to household income and
household net worth. Educational attainment was divided into five categories including less than
high school, completed high school, some college, completed college, and post-graduate
education. Self-reported poor health status reflects "fair" or "poor" health responses. Findings
confirm the robust relationships between household income (χ^2=36.81, df: 3.55, p<.001),
household net worth (χ^2=44.89, df: 3.19, p<.001), educational attainment (χ^2=36.65, df: 3.63,
p<.001) and self-reported poor health status as illustrated in Figure 5.3.

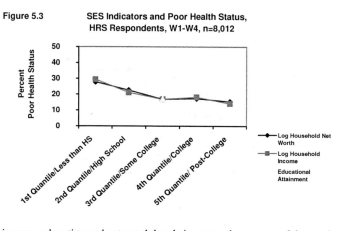

Figure 5.3   SES Indicators and Poor Health Status,
                    HRS Respondents, W1-W4, n=8,012

As income, education and net worth levels increase, the percent of those who report poor health
status decreases. As indicated in the Figure 5.3, the difference in respondents reporting poor
health status ranges from approximately 32% among those at the bottom of the hierarchy to an

average of 10% among those of the top, indicating a significantly monotonic association between SES and self-reported health status throughout the social spectrum.

Bivariate analyses are also conducted to examine whether SES influences mortality. Similar to poor health status, findings confirm that SES was also associated with mortality within the HRS dataset. Household income (χ^2= 20.34, df: 3.67, p<.001), household net worth (χ^2= 17.36, df: 3.58, p<.001), and educational attainment (χ^2= 7.11, df: 3.73, p<.001) are significantly and inversely associated with mortality as illustrated in Figure 5.4. Similar to the association between SES and health status, findings reveal both the magnitude and the consistency of the relationship between SES and mortality.

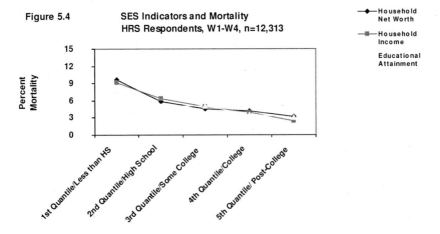

Figure 5.4   **SES Indicators and Mortality HRS Respondents, W1-W4, n=12,313**

Given that SES was clearly associated with health outcomes, the analysis proceeds to examine the next question:

Is SES associated with relative deprivation?

Figure 5.5 SES-Relative Deprivation Model

SES ——→ Relative Deprivation

To examine the relationship between SES and relative deprivation, relative income was calculated as the difference between a respondent's logged income and the logged median

45

income of one's respective zip code. This measure reflects income position with reference to what may be considered a community income norm. Since Wilkinson indicates that SES position influences health by causing dissatisfaction and stress, also referred to as "hierarchical stress," a measure of dissatisfaction with one's financial situation was used to represent this component of relative deprivation.

The correlation between absolute household income and relative household income (corr=.95) indicates a high degree of collinearity as illustrated in Figure 5.6.

Figure 5.6   Household Income and Relative Income
HRS Respondents, W1-W4, n=8,012

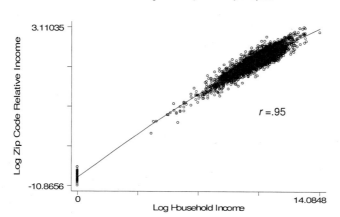

Since relative household income was derived from absolute household income, it was expected that these measures would be highly correlated. As household income increases, the higher the household income is in relation to their respective zip code median income level. Similarly, the higher the household net worth (χ^2= 34.72, df: 10.43, p<.001) and the higher the educational attainment (χ^2= 14.17, df: 9.41, p<.001), the higher the relative income position. Findings suggest that material advantage is positively linked to income position across all SES indicators. While findings indicate that SES was predictive of relative income, bivariate analyses are conducted to determine whether financial dissatisfaction was related to SES in a similar fashion. Household income (χ^2= 9.07, df: 12.33, p<.001), household net worth (χ^2= 23.81, df: 11.63, p<.001) and educational attainment (χ^2= 1.99, df: 11.77, p<.05) are found to be inversely associated with financial dissatisfaction.

46

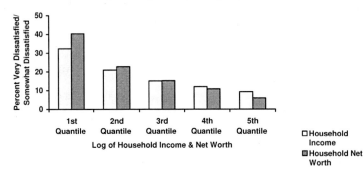

Figure 5.7   Household Net Worth, Household Income and Financial
                    Dissatisfaction, HRS Respondents, W1-W4, n=8,012

Figure 5.7 illustrates that as one proceeds from the lowest to the highest quintile of household net
worth and household income, the proportion of respondents who report "somewhat dissatisfied"
or "very dissatisfied" decreases, indicating that increasing net worth and household income
reduces financial dissatisfaction. Given that relative deprivation was associated with SES,
analyses are next conducted to examine the following question:

Is relative deprivation associated with health outcomes?

Figure 5.8 Relative Deprivation-Health Outcomes Model

Relative ⟶ Health Outcomes
Deprivation

Bivariate results indicate that financial dissatisfaction (χ^2= 15.22, df: 4.47, p<.001) and low
relative income at the zip code level (χ^2= 24.56, df: 3.30, p<.001) are positively associated with
poor health status. Figure 5.9 illustrates the two bivariate associations reflecting that the highest
proportion of respondents who report poor health status are included within the groups that
report "very dissatisfied," along with those within the 1st quintile or lowest level of relative
income.

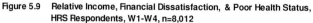

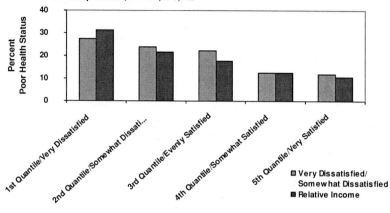

In summary, bivariate analyses demonstrate that 1) decreasing SES was directly associated with increasing relative deprivation and poor health outcomes, and 2) increasing relative deprivation was directly associated with poor health outcomes. While these findings demonstrate that relative deprivation was related to both SES and health, it remains unclear whether relative deprivation acts to significantly explain the relationship between SES and health. Thus, the next section of the analysis explores the following question:

Is relative deprivation, with respect to SES, predictive of health status, morbidity and mortality over time?

Figure 5.10 SES-Relative Deprivation-Health Outcomes Model

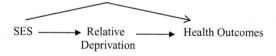

According to Wilkinson's hypothesis, relative income position, rather than absolute income level, is the causal factor driving the SES-health relationship in industrialized societies as shown in Figure 5.10 (Marmot and Wilkinson 2001). If this claim is valid, one would expect that those with similar absolute income levels, but different rank positions within an income

48

distribution (in relation to some referent category), would experience different health outcomes. Figure 5.11 illustrates two groups that differ with respect to median zip code income level. If rank position is operating as Wilkinson suggests, those at the bottom of a high-income group should experience higher levels of poor health outcomes as compared to those at the top of low-income group, regardless of absolute income level.

Figure 5.11 Wilkinson's Relative Deprivation Hypothesis

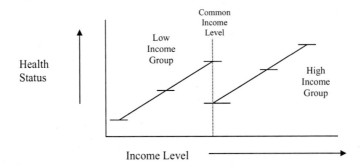

As a first step in testing this hypothesis, a strategic comparison of selected "rungs" of the income ladder was constructed by locating a situation where individuals have similar absolute income levels, but distinct rank positions in terms of household income to those around them. To compare income position within an income distribution with respect to absolute income, the zip code income distribution of HRS respondents was divided into 10 quantiles, from which the top and bottom 10% of the distribution are extracted. Although this comparison was limited to a small portion of the sample (20%), the stark contrast in relative and absolute income levels should enable one to demonstrate the differential health outcomes as described by Wilkinson. Following this strategic comparison, analyses are conducted within a multivariable context. Each of the two groups (high-income and low-income zip codes) are stratified into two relative income categories, low and high, based on each respondent's difference score from their respective zip code median income level, yielding a total four subgroups as indicated in Table 5.1. High relative income reflects those with incomes above the median income level for their respective zip code, and low relative income represents those whose incomes are below their median zip code level. Table 5.1 indicates the relative levels of health outcomes as would be predicted by Wilkinson's hypothesis. Rank position or being at the top of an income distribution, regardless of income level, should reduce relative deprivation, and thus, confer a health advantage as reflected in subgroups A and D.

Table 5.1 Predicted Proportion of Poor Health Outcomes		
	Low Relative Household Income	High Relative Household Income
High Income Zip Code Group	Subgroup A	Subgroup B
(Top 10% of Zip Code Median Income)	**Medium**	**Lowest**
Low Income Zip Code Group	Subgroup C	Subgroup D
(Bottom 10% of Zip Code Median Income)	**High**	**Low**

To validly compare predicted to actual values, actual mean zip code income levels and proportions of health outcomes are calculated for each of the four subgroups as shown in Table 5.2. Similar to the previous analyses, the sample was limited to those respondents who report good/very good/excellent health status and no life-threatening conditions at wave 1 (1992). Actual findings in Table 5.2 are compared to predicted proportions of health outcomes in Table 5.1. Comparison subgroups are shaded in grey for easy identification.

If one examines the proportions of health outcomes by zip code group alone, it's not surprising that those in the high-income groups experience lower proportions of poor health status, life-threatening conditions and death in comparison to the low- income groups, regardless of relative income level. Those doubly burdened by experiencing both low absolute and relative income, or being the poorest of the poor, report significantly high proportions of poor health outcomes with respect to health status (36.9%), having any life-threatening conditions (20.7%), and mortality (12%).

Recall that Wilkinson's relative deprivation hypothesis would predict a higher rate of poor health outcomes for those at the bottom of a high-income group as compared to those at the top of a low-income group. T-tests indicate that the comparison subgroups (Subgroups A and D) do not significantly differ in their mean income level ($p=.16$ for poor health status, $p=.70$ for having any life-threatening conditions, and $p= .21$ for mortality tables), suggesting that these subgroups are similar in terms of financial resources. With respect to poor health status, the percentage of those respondents at the top of the income hierarchy of a low-income zip code group (18.4%) was over one-third higher than for those at the bottom of a high-income zip code

50

group (11.7%). For having any life-threatening conditions, the percentage of respondents in the high relative income/low income zip code group (18.6%) was slightly higher than that of the low relative income/ high-income zip code group (16.9%). Similar to poor health status, the percentage of deaths among those at the top of a low-income zip code (6.2%) was over one-third higher than that of those at the bottom of a high-income zip code group (3.9%).

Table 5.2 Actual Proportions of Health Outcomes		
Poor Self-Rated Health (w1-w4, N=1,601) **(Limited to good health at w1)**	**Low Relative Household Income**	**High Relative Household Income**
High Income Zip Code Group	Subgroup A	Subgroup B
(Mean Income Level)	11.7%	6.1%
	(50,743K)	(139,857K)
	n=392	n=392
	Subgroup C	Subgroup D
Low Income Zip Code Group	36.9%	18.4%
(Mean Income Level)	(15,769K)	(52,952K)
	n=409	n=408
Having any Life-threatening Conditions (w1-w4, N=1,268) **(only no conditions at w1)**	Low Relative Income	High Relative Income
High Income Zip Code Group	Subgroup A	Subgroup B
(Mean Income Level)	16.9%	13.6%
	(51,311K)	(141,557K)
	n=289	n=332
	Subgroup C	Subgroup D
Low Income Zip Code Group	20.7%	18.6%
(Mean Income Level)	(16,610K)	(51,991K)
	n=319	n=328
Mortality (w1-w4, N=2,466)	Low Relative Income	High Relative Income
	Subgroup A	Subgroup B
High Income Zip Code Group	3.9%	1.8%
(Mean Income Level)	(45,845K)	(131,399K)
	n=616	n=613
	Subgroup C	Subgroup D
Low Income Zip Code Group	12%	6.2%
(Mean Income Level)	(11,489K)	(44,289K)
	n=620	n=617

Actual proportions of health outcomes indicate that the direction of the relative income effect was opposite to that of Wilkinson's hypothesis. Chi-square tests to determine whether the proportions of health outcomes are statistically different between comparison subgroups indicate that in the case of poor health status, proportions significantly differ, but in the opposite direction as to what Wilkinson's hypothesis would suggest ($\chi2 = 6.9$, $p<.01$). Proportions of having any life-threatening conditions ($\chi2 = .28$, $p=.59$) and mortality ($\chi2 = 3.3$, $p=.069$) do not significantly differ between comparison subgroups. Although Wilkinson's theory predicts that being at the top a low-income group results in better health outcomes, subgroup analyses do not lend support to this claim. Contrary to Wilkinson's theory, findings indicate that those at the bottom of a high-income group have significantly lower proportions of poor health status, while having any life-threatening conditions and mortality do not significantly differ.

In sum, actual health outcomes do not reflect predicted patterns of health outcomes. As such, results of the strategic informative comparisons do not lend support to Wilkinson's relative deprivation hypothesis. Multivariable analyses are now conducted to confirm the effect of relative deprivation in the simultaneous context of other variables.

Multivariable Analysis: the process of model development

To further investigate the role of relative deprivation, multivariable linear and logistic models are developed to uncover components of the SES-health association using progressive adjustment i.e., holding constant hypothesized mediators such as relative income difference and financial dissatisfaction in a sequential fashion (Mirowsky 1999; Susser 1973). Each model was examined with regard to significance of the variables being added, and the effect of the association between SES and health outcomes.

In the first phase of the analysis, linear regression models are developed to: 1) confirm the independent bivariate associations between SES, relative income and financial dissatisfaction, and 2) examine the conjoint SES effects on relative income and financial dissatisfaction while testing for potential confounding with demographic characteristics. Since the first component of Wilkinson's hypothesis indicates that relative income position causes financial dissatisfaction, linear regression models are then constructed to test whether relative income was predictive of financial dissatisfaction, with and without adjustment for demographic characteristics. The full model includes the following:

Financial Dissatisfaction $= b_0 + b1_{income} + b2_{education} + b3_{net\ worth} + b4_{relative\ income} + b5_{race/ethnicity} + b6_{age} + b7_{marital\ status} + \varepsilon$

In the next phase, models are developed to test the effects of relative income and financial dissatisfaction in the association between SES and health outcomes. Logistic regression models are first constructed to examine relative income position at three levels of geographic aggregation: the zip code, the county and state with respect to self-reported health status, having any life-threatening conditions, and mortality among men and women. The full model includes the following:

Logit (Poor Health Outcome) $= b_0 + b1_{income} + b2_{education} + b3_{net\ worth} + b4_{relative\ income} + b5_{race/ethnicity} + b6_{age} + b7_{marital\ status} + \varepsilon$

Similarly, models are then developed to examine the effects of financial dissatisfaction in the association between SES and health outcomes, controlling for other dissatisfaction indicators. Additional dissatisfaction variables, interpersonal dissatisfaction and dissatisfaction with life in general, are added to test whether financial dissatisfaction reflects a broader dissatisfaction in other life domains. The full model includes the following:

Logit (Poor Health Outcome) $= b_0 + b1_{income} + b2_{education} + b3_{net\ worth} + b4_{financial\ dissatisfaction} + b5_{interpersonal\ dissatisfaction} + b6_{life\ dissatisfaction} + b7_{race/ethnicity} + b8_{age} + b9_{marital\ status} + \varepsilon$

This strategy of building models by successively adding variables allows one to determine the direction and the magnitude of the effect of each hypothesized mediator in relation to the SES-health outcome association in question.

Is SES associated with relative deprivation?

The first hypothesis regarding relative deprivation puts forth the claim that decreasing socioeconomic status will be associated with decreasing relative income position and increasing financial dissatisfaction, and will not differ in terms of age, race/ethnicity, and marital status. SES may not necessarily be related to measures of relative advantage or deprivation since position within a reference group is independent of absolute measures of resources. That is to say, a teacher in a Mississippi school district who earns 40K/year may compare his income level to the state average income level for teachers, 30K, and feel relatively advantaged. In comparison, a teacher in New York earning 40K may feel relatively deprived when comparing themselves to a state average income for teachers at 50K. On the other hand, while SES isn't necessarily associated with relative position, the higher one's income, the higher one is from the reference standard. Furthermore, individuals tend to reside in areas that reflect their own demographic characteristics, thus, relative income may reflect absolute income.

To test this hypothesis, Table 5.3 presents the findings of linear regression models predicting relative income and financial dissatisfaction from SES indicators among women. SES indicators are examined separately to determine the independent effects of each component, and then combined into one model, with and without adjustment for potential confounders.

Model 1 through 4 reveal that while household income (b=.91, p<.001), educational attainment (b=.07, p<.001) and household net worth (b=.77, p<.001) are all highly significant and independent predictors of increasing relative income among women, the size of the coefficient for household income reflects its strong predictive effect. However, the coefficients for education and household net worth change to negative values when SES indicators are included in the model together. These changes are most likely the result of the high degree of collinearity between the SES indicators. After adjusting for potential confounders in Model 5, all SES indicators remain stable, demonstrating that demographic characteristics are not acting as confounders.

In terms of financial dissatisfaction among women, decreasing household income (b=-.22, p<.001), educational attainment (b=-.03, p<.05) and household net worth (b=-1.16, p<.001) are all highly significant and independent predictors of financial dissatisfaction among women. The full model (model 5) indicates that while decreasing household income and household net worth are significantly predictive of financial dissatisfaction, being younger and living without a partner also significantly influences the likelihood of financial dissatisfaction among women. Findings indicate that material disadvantage among women is linked to feelings of dissatisfaction with one's financial situation.

Table 5.3 Relative Income and Financial Dissatisfaction Regression Models for WOMEN; Limited to those with excellent/good health at W1

Covariates	Linear Regression used for outcome: Relative Income (Zip Code) (n=4,378)[c]					Linear Regression used for outcome: Financial Dissatisfaction (n=4,305)[c]				
	Model 1 Beta (SE)	Model 2 Beta (SE)	Model 3 Beta (SE)	Model 4 Beta (SE)	Model 5 Beta (SE)	Model 1 Beta (SE)	Model 2 Beta (SE)	Model 3 Beta (SE)	Model 4 Beta (SE)	Model 5 Beta (SE)
Log Household Income	.91† (.01)			.94† (.01)	.94† (.01)	-.22† (.03)			-.16† (.03)	-.12† (.03)
Education		.07† (.009)		-.03† (.004)	-.03† (.41)		-.03* (.01)		.02* (.01)	.02 (.01)
Log Household Net Worth			.77† (.09)	-.17† (.03)	-.17** (.03)			-1.16† (.08)	-1.04† (.08)	-.90† (.08)
Race/ Ethnicity										
White[a]					-.25† (.03)					-.198* (.09)
Hispanic[a]					-.21† (.04)					.003 (.13)
Other[a]					-.26† (.04)					-.19 (.16)
Age					.001 (.002)					-.03† (.007)
Married[b]					.05 (.02)					-.35† (.07)
R^2	.89†	.03†	.05†	.89†	.90†	.04†	.003*	.08†	.10†	.13†

[a] Compared to Blacks;
[b] Compared to never married, divorced, widowed, or separated   *p<.05, **p<.01, †p<.001
[c] Differences in sample size reflect financial dissatisfaction without imputations when used as DV

Similar to the results among women, household income (b=.87, p<.001), educational attainment (b=.07, p<.001) and household net worth (b=.81, p<.001) are all highly significant and independent predictors of increasing relative income among men as presented in Table 5.4. However, when all SES indicators are included into the model, the coefficients for education and net worth change to negative values. Adjustment for potential confounders does not appreciably change the effect sizes of the SES indicators, indicating that age, race/ethnicity and marital status do not mediate the SES-relative income relationship among men.

Table 5.4 Relative Income and Financial Dissatisfaction Regression Models for MEN Limited to those with excellent/good health at W1

	Linear Regression used for outcome: Relative Income (Zip Code) $(n=3,634)^{c}$					Linear Regression used for outcome: Financial Dissatisfaction $(n=3,378)^{c}$				
Covariates	Model 1 Beta (SE)	Model 2 Beta (SE)	Model 3 Beta (SE)	Model 4 Beta (SE)	Model 5 Beta (SE)	Model 1 Beta (SE)	Model 12 Beta (SE)	Model 3 Beta (SE)	Model 4 Beta (SE)	Model 5 Beta (SE)
Log Household Income	.87† (.02)			.91† (.01)	.91† (.01)	-.18† (.04)			-.11** (.04)	-.13** (.04)
Education		.07† (.006)		-.03† (.004)	-.03† (.004)		-.01 (.013)		.02 (.01)	.02 (.01)
Log Household Net Worth			.81† (.08)	-.09* (.04)	-.005 (.01)			-.93† (.13)	-.84† (.16)	-.80† (.14)
Race/ Ethnicity										
White[a]					-.24 † (.04)					.02 (.14)
Hispanic[a]					-21† (.05)					.11 (.20)
Other[a]					-.25** (.07)					.15 (.19)
Age					.006* (.002)					-.03** (.01)
Married[b]					.01 (.03)					.16 (.098)
R^2	.86†	.05†	.08†	.86†	.87†	.03†	.001	.06†	.07†	.11†

[a] Compared to Blacks;
[b] Compared to never married, divorced, widowed, or separated   *p<.05, ** p<.01, † p<.001
[c] Differences in sample size reflect financial dissatisfaction without imputations when used as DV

With regard to financial dissatisfaction among men, as household income (b= -.18, p<.001) and household net worth (b=-.93, p<.001) decreases, the degree of financial dissatisfaction significantly increases as shown in Table 5.4. As seen in previous analyses, the coefficient for educational attainment changes to a negative value and loses significance when all SES indicators are added as shown in model 4. Model 5 reveals the persistence of household income and household net worth to significantly predict financial dissatisfaction, adjusting for potential confounders. SES effects remain stable indicating that demographic characteristics do not fully explain the SES-financial dissatisfaction association. However, younger men are more likely to report financial dissatisfaction, controlling for SES.

In general, results of linear regression models for both men and women specify that decreasing SES was significantly associated with decreasing relative income and increasing financial dissatisfaction. Although several coefficient signs change when all SES indicators are included, models that examine SES indicators separately reveal a strong and significant predictive effect in the expected direction. These direct effects suggest that the change in coefficient sign was the result of collinearity among the SES indicators. Adjustment for potential confounders among men and women with respect to both relative income and financial dissatisfaction does not significantly reduce the SES effect, indicating that confounding was not a concern. Although findings show that SES was associated with relative income position and financial dissatisfaction, the next analysis sought to examine the following question:

Is relative income position associated with financial dissatisfaction?

The second hypothesis claims that low relative income position is associated with financial dissatisfaction, as theorizing by Wilkinson would lead us to expect. According to Wilkinson, one would expect low income position relative to a community norm to be positively associated with financial dissatisfaction, regardless of absolute material advantage. To test this hypothesis, a set of linear regression models is presented in Table 5.5. Estimates confirm the strong inverse association between SES and financial dissatisfaction as detailed in models 1 through 5. Model 6 reveals that having lower levels of income as compared to the median income level within one's zip code was significantly predictive of financial dissatisfaction among women, even after adjusting for demographic characteristics. Although taking account of socioeconomic status in model 7 renders relative income insignificant at the .05 level, closer examination reveals that the effect reaches significance at the .10 level (p=.084). Comparing models 5, 6 and 7, decreasing household net worth remains highly significant as a predictor of financial dissatisfaction whereas household income and education are reduced to nonsignificance. Findings suggests that although low-income position does not reach statistical significance in the full model, low-income position does appear to be associated with financial dissatisfaction among women, adjusting for SES. Across models, race, age and marital status persisted as significant predictors of financial dissatisfaction, controlling for SES. Black as compared to white women, younger women and women not living with a partner are more likely to report being dissatisfied with their financial situation.

Table 5.5	Financial Dissatisfaction Coefficients from Explanatory Models (W1-W4) Limited to those with excellent/good health at W1						
	WOMEN (n=4,305)						
Covariates	Model 1 Beta (SE)	Model 2 Beta (SE)	Model 3 Beta (SE)	Model 4 Beta (SE)	Model 5 Beta (SE)	Model 6 Beta (SE)	Model 7 Beta (SE)
Log Household Income	-.223† (.030)			-.157† (.026)	-.125† (.026)		.016 (.085)
Education		-.026* (.010)		.020* (.010)	.017 (.011)		.013 (.010)
Log Household Net Worth			-1.164† (.084)	-1.039† (.083)	-.895† (.078)		-.917† (.078)
Log Relative Income (Zip Code)						-.171† (.030)	-.149 (.086)
Race/ Ethnicity							
White [a]					-.198* (.089)	-.352† (.088)	-.237* (.096)
Hispanic [a]					.003 (.128)	-.105 (.137)	-.030 (.129)
Other [a]					-.187 (.158)	-.321* (.154)	-.226 (.164)
Age					-.032† (.007)	-.039† (.007)	-.032† (.007)
Married [b]					-.350† (.065)	-.438† (.066)	-.343† (.065)

Linear Regression used for outcome: Financial Dissatisfaction
[a] Compared to Blacks;
[b] Compared to never married, divorced, widowed, or separated   *p<.05, **p<.01, † p<.001

Given the weight of evidence concerning the economic disadvantage experienced by minority and single women, it was not surprising that financial dissatisfaction was more prevalent among these groups. One might expect that younger people would report less financial dissatisfaction assuming that their incomes are typically higher. However, results are consistent with previous research which also found that older people tend to be more satisfied with their financial situation despite lower incomes (Schieman 2001; Schieman, Van Gundy, and Taylor 2001).

Does relative income operate in a similar fashion among men? To explore this question, linear regression models predicting financial dissatisfaction are shown in Table 5.6.

Table 5.6	Financial Dissatisfaction Coefficients from Explanatory Models (W1-W4) Limited to those with excellent/good health at W1						
MEN *(n=3,378)*							
Covariates	Model 1 Beta (SE)	Model 2 Beta (SE)	Model 3 Beta (SE)	Model 4 Beta (SE)	Model 5 Beta (SE)	Model 6 Beta (SE)	Model 7 Beta (SE)
Log Household Income	-.182† (.038)			-.113* (.042)	-.134** (.038)		.217 (.118)
Education		-.012 (.014)		.020 (.015)	.019 (.015)		.009 (.012)
Log Household Net Worth			-.928† (.127)	-.845† (.156)	-.797† (.144)		-.837† (.140)
Log Relative Income (Zip Code)						-.238† (.042)	-.384** (.124)
Race/ Ethnicity							
White [a]					.017 (.142)	-.088 (.140)	-.074 (.126)
Hispanic [a]					.105 (.195)	.047 (.187)	.029 (.186)
Other [a]					.149 (.195)	.041 (.187)	.044 (.206)
Age					-.034** (.011)	-.043** (.013)	-.031** (.010)
Married [b]					.157 (.098)	.155 (.100)	.159 (.091)

Linear Regression used for outcome: Financial Dissatisfaction
[a] Compared to Blacks;
[b] Compared to never married, divorced, widowed, or separated   *p<.05, **p<.01, † p<.001

Models 1 through 4 indicate that while decreasing household income (b= -.182, p<.001) and household net worth (b= -.928, p<.001) are significantly predictive of financial dissatisfaction, educational attainment does not reach statistical significance. This finding may reflect the wage gap between men and women, controlling for educational attainment (Morris and Western 1999). Specifically, men continue to earn more income than women, even after adjusting for educational attainment. In contrast to the findings among women, low relative income position (b= -.384, p<.01) was significantly predictive of financial dissatisfaction in addition to decreasing household net worth (b= -.837, p<.001) and younger age (b= -.031, p<.01) as indicated in model 7. Race and marital status were not associated with financial dissatisfaction among men.

Overall, findings suggest that low relative income position, adjusting for SES, was predictive of financial dissatisfaction. In other words, those at the bottom of an income distribution are more likely to be dissatisfied with their financial situation, regardless of absolute income or net worth. While results indicate that this association was stronger for men than for women, findings lend support to Wilkinson's premise that relative income position produces negative psychosocial effects such as financial dissatisfaction. While SES was found to be associated with both relative income and financial dissatisfaction, and relative income was found to be predictive of financial dissatisfaction, the final analysis sought to answer the following question:

Does relative deprivation mediate the SES-health association?

The third hypothesis to be tested indicates that relative deprivation will significantly reduce the size of the direct SES effect on health outcome variables, and thus, mediate or explain this association. To evaluate this hypothesis, models are constructed to test the general effect of SES on health outcomes, and the independent effects of relative deprivation as measured by relative income and financial dissatisfaction. Given that the relationship between income and health outcomes is often found to include a curved component, squared income terms were added to regression models to determine the functional form of the relationship between health outcomes, income, and net worth. If squared terms of independent variables are found to be significantly associated with an outcome variable, it suggests that the form of the relationship includes a curvature effect in addition to the linear relationship. Although the squared term for household income was found to be significantly associated with self-reported health status, inclusion of the squared term did not change any of the findings. Financial dissatisfaction was also determined to be linearly related to health outcomes. Thus, squared terms are not included within any of the analyses. Logistic regression results for men and women are presented sequentially by health outcome. Since logistic regression coefficients are not easy to interpret apart from the sign and significance, odds ratios and their respective confidence intervals are also indicated for selected analyses.

60

Self-Rated Health Status

This group of models includes logistic regression results of poor health status on SES, relative income at the zip code level, and financial dissatisfaction at wave 4 among women who reported good/very good/excellent health at wave 1. The estimates in Table 5.7 (models 1 and 2) confirm the robust inverse relationship between household income (b= -.196, p<.001), educational attainment (b= -.165, p<.001), household net worth (b= -.786, p<.05), and poor health status, with and without adjustment for age, marital status, and race/ethnicity. The odds of reporting poor health status was significantly reduced as educational attainment (OR=.847, CI: .811, .885), household income (OR=.822, CI: .756, .893), and household net worth (OR=.455, CI: .246, .840) increases. For example, the odds of reporting poor self-rated health are 1.5 times larger for women in the 10th percentile of household income as compared to women within the 90th percentile, holding other SES indicators constant. Comparing women high school graduates to women who graduated college, the odds of reporting poor self-rated health are approximately doubled (2.0) for high school graduates. In terms of household net worth, women in the 10th percentile experience 1.5 times the odds of reporting poor health status as compared to women within the 90th percentile of household net worth.

Model 3 reveals the role of relative income in that the lower a respondent was from the median income level within their respective zip code, the more likely they are to report poor health status (b= -.233, p<.001, OR=.792, CI: .724, .867), adjusting for demographic variables. To determine whether relative income partially explains socioeconomic variations in women's poor health status, the association between SES and health status must be examined with and without adjustment for relative income. If adjustment for relative income significantly reduces (reduces the beta coefficient more than 10%) the association between SES and poor health status, then it helps mediate or explain the association (Baron and Kenny 1986). In addition, low relative income must be significantly associated with poor health outcomes, controlling for absolute income.

Model 4 indicates that relative income loses significance as a predictor of poor health status when SES indicators are added to the model. Comparing models 2 and 4, household income loses significance and relative income does not remain significantly associated with poor health status among women within the full model (Model 4). Thus, relative income position does not mediate the association between SES and poor health status among women.

61

Table 5.7   **Poor Self-Rated Health Status Coefficients from Explanatory Models (W1-W4) Limited to those with excellent/good health at W1**

WOMEN *(n=4,378)*

Covariates	Model 1 Beta (SE)	Model 2 Beta (SE)	Model 3 Beta (SE)	Model 4 Beta (SE)	Model 5 Beta (SE)	Model 6 Beta (SE)	Model 7 Beta (SE)
Log Household Income	-.196† (.041)	-.182† (.040)		-.153 (.179)		-.153† (.039)	-.154† (.038)
Education	-.165† (.022)	-.155† (.022)		-.155† (.023)		-.160† (.023)	-.162† (.023)
Log Household Net Worth	-.786* (.306)	-.588 (.297)		-.594 (.304)		-.232 (.274)	-.233 (.271)
Log Relative Income (Zip Code)			-.233† (.045)	-.031 (.186)			
Financial Dissatisfaction					.347† (.044)	.305† (.045)	.256† (.052)
Interpersonal Dissatisfaction							.022 (.024)
Life Dissatisfaction							.136 (.085)
Race/ Ethnicity							
White [a]		-.340* (.146)	-.579† (.136)	-.348* (.157)	-.463** (.137)	-.292* (.143)	-.306* (.141)
Hispanic [a]		.226 (.264)	.596* (.255)	.219 (.273)	.681** (.235)	.251 (.255)	.272 (.253)
Other [a]		-.032 (.412)	-.300 (.462)	-.039 (.425)	-.169 (.467)	.014 (.432)	.026 (.424)
Age		-.034* (.017)	-.028 (.017)	-.035* (.017)	-.012 (.018)	-.025 (.018)	-.025 (.018)
Married [b]		-.184 (.137)	-.221 (.136)	-.182 (.138)	-.180 (.127)	-.072 (.137)	.050 (.139)

Logistic Regression used for outcome: Self-Rated Health
[a] Compared to Blacks;
[b] Compared to never married, divorced, widowed, or separated   *p<.05, **p<.01, † p<.001

Model 5 reveals that high financial dissatisfaction (b=.347, p<.001) was significantly predictive of poor health status when examining its direct effects, or adjusting for potential confounders. In other terms, the more financially dissatisfied a respondent was, the higher the odds of reporting poor health status (OR=1.415, CI: 1.296, 1.543). Specifically, the odds of reporting poor self-reported health are over three times greater for women who report "very dissatisfied" as compared to women who report "very satisfied" with their financial situation. As indicated previously, additional dissatisfaction indicators are added to test whether financial dissatisfaction was a function of being generally dissatisfied, or feeling dissatisfied within other life domains. However, financial dissatisfaction was found to persist as a highly significant predictor of poor health status (b= .305, p<.001), even after controlling for all SES indicators, demographic characteristics, and other dissatisfaction indicators as represented in the full model (model 7). Furthermore, the addition of financial dissatisfaction reduces the income effect by 15% (from -.182 to -.153) as shown in model 6. Low educational attainment and being black, as compared to white, remains significantly associated with poor health status among women. Therefore, evidence suggests that financial dissatisfaction mediates some portion of the association between SES and poor health status among women.

Are associations between SES, relative income, and financial dissatisfaction the same in men as they are in women? To explore this question, logistic regression analyses are repeated for men, mirroring the analytic strategy for women. Findings presented in Table 5.8 reflect the significantly predictive effects of decreasing household income (b= -.233, p<.01, OR=.822, CI: .811, .885), educational attainment (b= -.150, p<.001, OR=.847, CI: .756, .892), and net worth (b= -.594, p<.05, OR=.445, CI: .246, .840) on poor health status. Similar to the odds for women, the odds of reporting poor self-rated health are 50% higher for men within the 10th percentile of household income as compared to men within the 90th percentile, holding other SES indicators constant. Moreover, a male high school graduate was estimated to experience an 80% increase in the odds of reporting poor health as compared to a male college graduate, holding other SES indicators constant. Model 3 indicates that being at the bottom of one's income group (b= -.256, p<.001) and identifying as a black man significantly increases the likelihood of reporting poor health status. In terms of the odds of reporting poor health status among men, the higher one was in relation to their zip code income group (OR= .774, CI: .675, 886) and being white, as compared to black, (OR= .443, CI: .215, .912) significantly reduces one's odds of reporting poor health. However, adding relative income into the full model (model 4) renders relative income insignificant as a predictor of poor health status and changes the sign of the coefficient from negative to positive (b= .254). To the extent that relative income has any effect at all, it was in a direction opposite to that predicted by relative deprivation. Comparing model 2 and 4, relative income reduces the direct effects of education (4%) and net worth (25%), while increasing the direct effect of household income considerably (57%). Thus, relative income position may not be considered to act as a mediator in the SES-health status association among men.

Table 5.8   Poor Self-Rated Health Status Coefficients from Explanatory Models (W1-W4) Limited to those with excellent/good health at W1)

	MEN (n=3,634)						
Covariates	Model 1 Beta (SE)	Model 2 Beta (SE)	Model 3 Beta (SE)	Model 4 Beta (SE)	Model 5 Beta (SE)	Model 6 Beta (SE)	Model 7 Beta (SE)
Log Household Income	-.233** (.082)	-.182** (.063)		-.419** (.151)		-.165* (.062)	-.178** (.066)
Education	-.150† (.020)	-.150† (.022)		-.144† (.023)		-.153† (.022)	-.158 (.023)
Log Household Net Worth	-.594* (.257)	-.481 (.246)		-.444 (.246)		-.332 (.236)	-.299 (.240)
Log Relative Income (Zip Code)			-.256† (.067)	.254 (.139)			
Financial Dissatisfaction					.192** (.061)	.152* (.059)	.076 (.078)
Interpersonal Dissatisfaction							.041 (.029)
Life Dissatisfaction							.142 (.105)
Race/ Ethnicity							
White [a]		-.465 (.372)	-.814* (.361)	-.396 (.364)	-.829* (.385)	-.481 (.390)	-.509 (.375)
Hispanic [a]		-.325 (.460)	-.046 (.414)	-.268 (.460)	-.020 (.436)	-.350 (.476)	-.384 (.476)
Other [a]		-.140 (.513)	-.631 (.499)	-.073 (.514)	-.686 (.501)	-.169 (.516)	-.185 (.513)
Age		.005 (.017)	.016 (.017)	.004 (.018)	.026 (.018)	.009 (.019)	.013 (.018)
Married [b]		-.463* (.226)	-.409 (.223)	-.462* (.225)	-.587* (.236)	-.490* (.231)	-.389 (.204)

Logistic Regression used for outcomes: Self-Rated Health
[a] Compared to Blacks;
[b] Compared to never married, divorced, widowed, or separated   *p<.05, **p<.01, †p<.001

Models 5 and 6 specify that financial dissatisfaction (b= -.152, p<.05) was a significant predictor of poor health status among men, controlling for SES indicators and demographic characteristics. The odds of reporting poor health status are elevated by 84% among men who report being "very dissatisfied" with their financial situation. Comparing models 2 and 6 shows

64

that financial dissatisfaction persists as a significant predictor of poor health status (b= .152, p< .05), despite adjustment for SES and demographic characteristics, and substantially reduces the effect of household net worth (31%). In contrast to the effect of financial dissatisfaction among women, adjusting for the additional dissatisfaction indicators renders financial dissatisfaction insignificant among men within the full model (model 7). To determine whether financial dissatisfaction significantly differs by gender, an interaction term was included in a model not stratified by gender. The financial dissatisfaction/gender interaction term was not found to be significantly different (results not shown). Thus, findings suggest that the effect of financial dissatisfaction was weaker with respect to self-reported health status among men.

In general, results indicate that relative income position measured at the zip code level does not mediate the association between SES and poor health status for either women or men. Without controlling for household income, the measure of relative income was in large part a measure of household income. While relative income does not appear to be independently important in the association between SES and health status, it was shown to be predictive of financial dissatisfaction in the predicted direction. Financial dissatisfaction, however, was shown to be a strong and persistent predictor of poor health status. Although controlling for additional dissatisfaction indicators reduces the effect of financial dissatisfaction among men, evidence suggests that financial dissatisfaction may play a role in explaining a portion of the association between SES and poor health status.

Having Any Life-threatening Conditions

The general pattern of socioeconomic disadvantage in relation to poor health status was also observed when we turn our attention to having life-threatening conditions.
To examine the relationship of having any life-threatening conditions to SES, zip code level-relative income, and demographic variables, logistic regression analyses are conducted for women who report no life-threatening conditions at baseline (wave 1). Like the estimates shown in Table 5.7, models 1 and 2 in Table 5.9 show that SES significantly influences the onset of having any life-threatening conditions among women.

Decreasing household income (b= -.107, p<.01), low educational attainment (b= -.073, p<.001), decreasing household net worth (b= -.665, p<.05) and low relative income position (b= -.130, p<.01) are significantly predictive of having any life-threatening conditions, with and without adjustment for demographic variables. Increasing household income (OR=.887, CI: .819, .960), educational attainment (OR=.933, CI: .903, .963), net worth (OR=.521, CI: .287, .947) and relative income position (OR=.859, CI: .796, .927) independently reduce the odds of having any life-threatening conditions among women.

Table 5.9 Having Any Life-threatening Conditions Coefficients from Explanatory Models (W1-W4) Limited to those without any conditions at W1

Covariates	WOMEN (n=3,964)						
	Model 1 Beta (SE)	Model 2 Beta (SE)	Model 3 Beta (SE)	Model 4 Beta (SE)	Model 5 Beta (SE)	Model 6 Beta (SE)	Model 7 Beta (SE)
Log Household Income	-.120** (.040)	-.107** (.039)		-.345 (.184)		-.097* (.040)	-.097* (.041)
Education	-.069† (.016)	-.073† (.019)		-.067** (.019)		-.073† (.018)	-.075† (.019)
Log Household Net Worth	-.651* (.298)	-.665* (.312)		-.617 (.318)		-.578 (.306)	-.577 (.305)
Log Relative Income (Zip Code)			-.130** (.036)	.247 (.181)			
Financial Dissatisfaction					.138† (.037)	.080* (.039)	.038 (.044)
Interpersonal Dissatisfaction							.035 (.031)
Life Dissatisfaction							.064 (.097)
Race/ Ethnicity							
White [a]		.052 (.126)	-.238 (.121)	.102 (.128)	-.182 (.127)	-.030 (.128)	-.028 (.125)
Hispanic [a]		-.245 (.228)	-.045 (.216)	-.199 (.225)	-.012 (.211)	-.245 (.229)	-.245 (.231)
Other [a]		-.084 (.354)	-.292 (.367)	-.024 (.367)	-.251 (.364)	-.063 (.352)	-.038 (.349)
Age		.030 (.017)	.029 (.017)	.030 (.017)	.038* (.017)	.033 (.017)	.032 (.017)
Married [b]		-.069 (.120)	-.133 (.120)	-.078 (.119)	-.152 (.123)	-.043 (.118)	-.023 (.114)

Logistic Regression used for outcomes: Having Any Life-threatening Conditions
[a] Compared to Blacks;
[b] Compared to never married, divorced, widowed, or separated   *p<.05, **p<.01, †p<.001

For instance, the difference in the odds of having any life-threatening conditions was approximately 30% higher for women in the 10th percentile of household income as compared to women within the 90th percentile. Similarly, having any life-threatening conditions among women was 1.3 times greater for high school graduates as compared to college graduates. Yet, once all indicators are included in the model, relative income loses significance and the sign of the coefficient changes to a positive value (b=.247). Similar to its role in the health status analysis, relative income does not substantially reduce the education and net worth effects, but leads to an increase in the direct effect of income. Results do not indicate that relative income mediates the SES effect on having any life-threatening conditions among women.

Model 6 shows that after adjusting for SES indicators and demographic characteristics, financial dissatisfaction persists as significantly associated with having any life-threatening condition (b= .080, p<.05). Furthermore, the income effect was reduced by approximately 10% when financial dissatisfaction was added into the model. Taken together, findings are suggestive of mediation. However, the addition of the other dissatisfaction indicators renders financial dissatisfaction insignificant and the SES effects remain stable (model 7). In contrast to the evidence shown for the SES-health status association, findings do not indicate financial dissatisfaction acts as a mediator in the association between SES and having any life-threatening conditions among women.

Models are presented in Table 5.10 to examine how relative deprivation operates with respect to having any life-threatening conditions among men who report no conditions at baseline. Interestingly, decreasing household income (b= .120, p<.05, OR=.888, CI: .807, .978) and increasing age are significantly associated with having any conditions among men, but neither educational attainment nor household net worth are independent significant predictors of conditions among men. For example, the odds of having any life-threatening conditions are 26% higher for men in the 10th percentile of household income as compared to men within the 90th percentile. Similar to findings among women, relative income significantly predicts having any conditions in the correct direction when adjusting for demographic characteristics, but it loses significance and the coefficient changes to a positive value when SES indicators are included as shown in model 4.

To discern whether financial dissatisfaction acts as a mediator, models 5 through 7 are compared. Results reveal that decreasing household income (b= -.108, p<.05), increasing financial dissatisfaction (b= .128, p<.05), and increasing age (b= .055, p<.01) significantly predict having any conditions among men, controlling for race/ethnicity, marital status and other dissatisfaction indicators. In other terms, the odds of having any conditions are 70% higher for men who report "very dissatisfied" as compared to men who report "very satisfied" with their financial situation, holding demographic and other dissatisfaction indicators constant. In addition, financial dissatisfaction substantially reduces the effect of household income (59%) and net worth (12%) when it was included in model 6, indicating that financial dissatisfaction may be mediating a portion of the association between SES and having any life-threatening conditions among men.

Table 5.10 Having Any Life-threatening Conditions Coefficients from Explanatory Models (W1-W4) Limited to those without any conditions at W1							
MEN (n=3,111)							
Covariates	Model 1 Beta (SE)	Model 2 Beta (SE)	Model 3 Beta (SE)	Model 4 Beta (SE)	Model 5 Beta (SE)	Model 6 Beta (SE)	Model 7 Beta (SE)
Log Household Income	-.118* (.048)	-.120* (.050)		-.268 (.188)		-.109* (.050)	-.108* (.050)
Education	-.001 (.016)	.001 (.017)		.003 (.018)		-.001 (.018)	.002 (.018)
Log Household Net Worth	-.253 (.189)	-.366 (.203)		-.343 (.199)		-.302 (.206)	-.313 (.205)
Log Relative Income (Zip Code)			-.124* (.051)	.159 (.193)			
Financial Dissatisfaction					.123* (.052)	.089 (.053)	.128* (.055)
Interpersonal Dissatisfaction							-.030 (.025)
Life Dissatisfaction							-.054 (.095)
Race/ Ethnicity							
White [a]		.002 (.180)	-.087 (.174)	.035 (.189)	-.064 (.177)	.022 (.182)	.050 (.180)
Hispanic [a]		-.340 (.264)	-.347 (.266)	-.317 (.264)	-.308 (.268)	-.324 (.268)	-.290 (.263)
Other [a]		-.178 (.456)	-.290 (.448)	-.138 (.470)	-.297 (.462)	-.172 (.462)	-.142 (.463)
Age		.053* (.020)	.052** (.019)	.052* (.020)	.058** (.019)	.056** (.020)	.055** (.019)
Married [b]		.171 (.180)	.136 (.183)	.165 (.181)	.055 (.179)	.173 (.180)	.121 (.188)
Logistic Regression used for outcomes: Having Any Life-threatening Conditions [a] Compared to Blacks; [b] Compared to never married, divorced, widowed, or separated *p<.05, **p<.01, †p<.001							

68

In sum, findings indicate that relative income does not mediate the association between SES and having any life-threatening conditions for either women or men. However, evidence suggests that financial dissatisfaction mediates some portion of this relationship among men.

All-Cause Mortality

Using the same strategy of showing the separate and conjoint effects of SES, relative income, and financial dissatisfaction, the subsequent analyses examine whether relative deprivation mediates the relationship between SES and mortality. This sample was not limited to either those who report good health status or those without any life-threatening conditions. Rather, this analysis includes the larger sample in an effort to take account of those processes that are thought to contribute to early death.

Logistic regression models examining mortality among women at wave 4 (1998) is presented in Table 5.11. Decreasing household income (b= -.267, p< .001) and net worth (b= -1.25, p< .05) persist as significant predictors of mortality. Alternatively, increasing household income (OR=.766, CI: .663, .884) and net worth (OR=.286, CI: .089, .913) significantly reduce the odds of death among women. For example, the difference in the odds of death for women in the 10th percentile of household income and net worth are 80% higher as compared to women within the 90th percentile, holding other SES indicators constant. When demographic characteristics are added into the model, race/ethnicity and age persist as significantly associated with the likelihood of death across all models. Results reveal that black women as compared to whites and Hispanics are at a significantly higher risk for death. As would be expected, older age was also predictive of death.

Model 3 indicates that decreasing income position (b= -.252, p<.01) in relation to one's respective zip code median income level was significantly associated with mortality, adjusting for demographic characteristics. Like the previous analyses, relative income loses significance and the sign of the coefficient changes to a positive value when SES indicators are included as shown in model 4, while decreasing household income and net worth, as well as being black and older persist as significantly predictive of mortality. Increasing financial dissatisfaction (b= .225, p<.01, OR=1.25, CI: 1.09, 1.43) was significantly associated with mortality, adjusting for demographic characteristics in model 5. If we compare the opposite ends of the financial

69

dissatisfaction scale, the odds of dying for women who reported being "very dissatisfied" are approximately 2.5 times the odds of dying for women who reported being "very satisfied."

Table 5.11 Mortality Coefficients from Explanatory Models (W1-W4)							
Women (n=6,582)							
Covariates	Model 1 Beta (SE)	Model 2 Beta (SE)	Model 3 Beta (SE)	Model 4 Beta (SE)	Model 5 Beta (SE)	Model 6 Beta (SE)	Model 7 Beta (SE)
Log Household Income	-.267† (.072)	-.210* (.092)		-.453* (.214)		-.175 (.103)	-.176 (.104)
Education	-.040 (.021)	-.047 (.023)		-.042 (.024)		-.045 (.023)	-.044 (.023)
Log Household Net Worth	-1.252* (.581)	-1.240* (.562)		-1.191* (.554)		-1.078 (.023)	-1.077 (.562)
Log Relative Income (Zip Code)			-.252** (.076)	.259 (.189)			
Financial Dissatisfaction					.225** (.066)	.138 (.077)	.113 (.077)
Interpersonal Dissatisfaction							-.010 (.045)
Life Dissatisfaction							.103 (.110)
Race/ Ethnicity							
White [a]		-.391* (.171)	-.622** (.180)	-.322 (.178)	-.520** (.178)	-.352* (.169)	-.370* (.171)
Hispanic [a]		-.780** (.241)	-.677** (.230)	-.736** (.245)	-.644* (.233)	-.768** (.242)	-.763** (.241)
Other [a]		.153 (.343)	-.020 (.331)	.204 (.353)	.030 (.323)	.187 (.341)	.188 (.340)
Age		.070* (.031)	.067* (.031)	.070* (.031)	.081* (.031)	.075* (.032)	.074* (.033)
Married [b]		-.109 (.188)	-.228 (.198)	-.118 (.190)	-.255 (.175)	-.058 (.183)	-.042 (.183)
Logistic Regression used for outcomes: All-Cause Mortality [a] Compared to Blacks; [b] Compared to never married, divorced, widowed, or separated *p<.05, **p<.01, †p<.001							

Although financial dissatisfaction was a strong independent predictor of mortality, the inclusion of SES indicators and additional dissatisfaction indicators in the subsequent models (models 6 and 7) renders financial dissatisfaction statistically insignificant. As such, results do not indicate that either relative income position or financial dissatisfaction mediates the SES-mortality association among women.

The final analysis examining relative deprivation replicates the previous analytic strategy to determine the SES effect on mortality among men. Logistic regression models 1 and 2 in Table 5.12 reflect the strong association between decreasing household income (b= -.408, p<.001, OR=.664, CI: .569, .775) and mortality among men, adjusting for demographic characteristics.

Table 5.12 Mortality Coefficients from Explanatory Models (W1-W4)							
Men (n=5,731)							
Covariates	Model 1 Beta (SE)	Model 2 Beta (SE)	Model 3 Beta (SE)	Model 4 Beta (SE)	Model 5 Beta (SE)	Model 6 Beta (SE)	Model 7 Beta (SE)
Log Household Income	-.463† (.074)	-.408† (.077)		-.691† (.159)		-.349† (.074)	-.340† (.075)
Education	-.016 (.023)	-.025 (.025)		-.019 (.024)		-.028 (.024)	-.026 (.024)
Log Household Net Worth	-.249 (.329)	-.392* (.359)		-.347 (.358)		-.192 (.332)	-.204 (.326)
Log Relative Income (Zip Code)			-.405† (.077)	.305** (.177)			
Financial Dissatisfaction					.279† (.050)	.194† (.045)	.161** (.055)
Interpersonal Dissatisfaction							-.054* (.024)
Life Dissatisfaction							.248* (.098)
Race/ Ethnicity							
White [a]		-.246 (.203)	-.468* (.207)	-.178 (.199)	-.399 (.200)	-.205 (.202)	-.256 (.204)
Hispanic [a]		-1.135** (.362)	-1.107** (.349)	-1.094** (.360)	-.996** (.332)	-1.107** (.356)	-1.181** (.360)
Other [a]		-.047 (.542)	-.265 (.554)	.0218 (.543)	-.210 (.546)	-.034 (.550)	-.094 (.549)
Age		.093† (.016)	.096† (.016)	.092† (.017)	.113† (.018)	.098† (.017)	.099† (.017)
Married [b]		-.147 (.173)	-.212 (.177)	-.153 (.171)	-.392* (.174)	-.126 (.175)	-.117 (.188)
Logistic Regression used for outcomes: All-Cause Mortality [a] Compared to Blacks; [b] Compared to never married, divorced, widowed, or separated *p<.05, **p<.01, †p<.001							

The odds of a man in the 10th percentile of household income are 2.5 times greater than men within the 90th percentile, holding other SES indicators constant. Race/ethnicity and age persist as important influences for early death given that black men, as compared to Hispanic men, and older men are at increased risk for death.

Model 3 indicates that low relative income position was significantly predictive of mortality among men, even after adjusting for demographic characteristics. Similar to previous results, the strong influence of each of the SES indicators acts to change the sign of the relative income coefficient (b= .305, p<.01), however, relative income remains significantly associated with mortality among men as shown in model 4. There was a slight reduction in the effect of net worth (11%) on mortality when relative income was added, suggesting relative income may be mediating a small portion of the SES-mortality association among men. Black men, as compared to Hispanic men, are much more likely to die by wave 4 (b=-1.094, p<.01). Increasing age was also highly associated with death (b= .092, p<.001).

Models 5 through 7 reveal the strong and persistent influence of financial dissatisfaction on mortality among men. Decreasing household income (b= -.340, p<.001, OR=.711, CI: .612, .826) and increasing financial dissatisfaction (b= .161, p<.01, OR=1.174, CI: 1.05, 1.31) significantly predict mortality, even after adjustment for additional dissatisfaction indicators. In terms of odds of death among men, those in the 10th percentile of household income are twice as likely to die as those men within the 90th income percentile category. Reporting "very dissatisfied" with their financial situation increases a man's odds of death by 90%, as compared with men who reported being "very satisfied", adjusting for demographic, dissatisfaction, and SES indicators. Comparing models 2 and 6, Black men, as compared to Hispanic men, and increasing age persist in the full model as significant factors associated with mortality, despite adjusting for financial dissatisfaction and SES.

Summary of Findings

Wilkinson's hypothesis posits that relative deprivation is the primary mechanism through which SES influences health outcomes within industrialized societies. Specifically, relative income position leads to negative psychosocial consequences such as financial dissatisfaction that, in turn, result in poor health outcomes. Table 5.13 summarizes the findings.

Table 5.13 Summary of Relative Deprivation Findings		
Strategic Comparison Test	**Absolute or Relative?**	**Statistically significant?**
SRH	Absolute higher than relative	Groups significantly differ in favor of absolute
Conditions	Absolute higher than relative	No significant difference
Mortality	Absolute higher than relative	No significant difference

Multivariable Regression Models	**WOMEN**	**MEN**
SES→ Relative Income	**Positively associated?**	
Household Income	Yes	Yes
Household Net Worth	Yes	Yes
Education	Yes	Yes
SES → Financial Dissatisfaction	**Negatively associated?**	
Household Income	Yes	Yes
Household Net Worth	Yes	Yes
Education	Yes	Yes
Relative Income → Financial Dissatisfaction	**Negatively associated?**	
	Yes ($p<.10$)	Yes

SES→ Relative Deprivation→ Health Outcomes	**Does Mediation Occur?**	
SES→Financial Dissatisfaction→SRH	Yes	Yes
SES→Financial Dissatisfaction→Conditions	Yes	Yes ($p<.10$)
SES→Financial Dissatisfaction→Mortality	Yes ($p<.10$)	Yes
SES→Relative Income→SRH	No	No
SES→Relative Income→Conditions	No	No
SES→Relative Income→Mortality	No	Yes

Although the strategic comparison findings suggest that absolute, rather than relative, income strongly shapes health outcomes, the multivariable models provide a fair amount of compelling evidence which lend support to Wilkinson's hypothesis. First, all SES indicators are significantly associated with relative position among women and men in the expected direction (positively associated). Similarly, all SES indicators are significantly and inversely associated with financial dissatisfaction among women and men.

Secondly, relative income was found to be inversely associated with financial dissatisfaction adjusting for SES among women at the trend level (p< .10), and persists as a significant predictor among men, holding SES constant. In addition, relative income position was found to be independently associated with both SES and health outcomes among women and men in the expected direction.

Lastly, results suggest that financial dissatisfaction mediates a portion of the SES-health association. While relative income position does not meet the criteria for mediation, financial dissatisfaction was found to reduce SES effects, and persist as a significant predictor of health outcomes at or below the .05 significance level in four of the six tests for mediation. The remaining two tests reveal significance at the trend level (p<.10). Of the 27 gender-specific multivariable models tested, 22 models (81%) provide empirical evidence which support Wilkinson's hypothesis.

Additional Geographic Aggregations

While the selection of a reference group has been typically based on geographic proximity (Singer 1981), there is little consensus with regard to which geographic aggregation approximates the most salient social comparison referent. For this study, zip code is chosen as the focus for examining relative deprivation because of its comparability to a "neighborhood." However, questions remain. Do people compare themselves to those within their neighborhood such as a zip code area, to a broader community standard such as a county, or to does this comparison process operate at the state level? To examine the possible variations between geographic reference standards, relative deprivation analyses (identical to those conducted for zip code relative income) are conducted using two alternate geographic aggregations: US county and state. Tables presenting the results of multivariable analyses are included in Appendix 1 and 2.

In general, results are similar to those found for relative income measured at the zip code level. Increasing SES was significantly and positively associated with relative income, and decreasing relative income was inversely related to health outcomes. However, relative income was not found to mediate the SES-health association at either the state or county level. Overall, the role of relative income was not found to differ across geographic aggregations.

Chapter VI

SES, Resource Utilization, and Health Outcomes

This chapter discusses the results of analyses testing the hypotheses derived from the Fundamental Cause idea. This theoretical perspective indicates that resource utilization drives the persistence of the SES-health gradient through a process of leveraging absolute resources in an incalculable number of ways which translate incrementally into health advantages throughout the social hierarchy (Link and Phelan 1996).

Figure 6.1 illustrates the relationship between resources, in the form of money, knowledge, power, prestige, and social connectedness, and one's ability to reduce one's risk of risk within a complex web of exposure to health threats as specified by the Fundamental Cause hypothesis. Resources are thought to facilitate the adoption or employment of risk-reduction and health promotion strategies through individual and contextual processes. The Fundamental Cause perspective stresses the importance of absolute resources as the primary, though not the only, mechanism through which SES shapes health and longevity.

Figure 6.1 Fundamental Cause Hypothesis

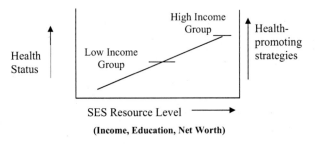

If resource utilization partially mediates the association between SES and health, the same conditions for mediation must be met as was indicated in the previous chapter. Specifically, the SES-health relationship will be partially explained or accounted for by the Health-Related Resource Index (HRRI). Results must indicate that compared with those with low resource utilization, those who report increasing resource utilization experience better health outcomes. In addition, the association between SES and health outcomes should be reduced after adjustment for resource utilization. Alternatively, if controlling resource utilization fails to reduce the SES-health association or if resource utilization is not correlated to health when SES is controlled, mediation cannot be inferred.

While the hypotheses indicate that health-related resource utilization will partially mediate the SES-health association, it should be emphasized that this dynamic process as measured here may mediate the relationship at this time in history, but it probably didn't in the past and may not in the future. This operationalization is linked to the major causes of disability and death at present, but as time goes on, society will face new health threats that will require different resource items to be leveraged to gain a health advantage. Nonetheless, the items included in the HRRI are mediators that Fundamental Cause would specify and not the mediators that the Relative Deprivation/Hierarchy Stress perspective would specify.

Figure 6.2 Fundamental Cause Explanatory Model

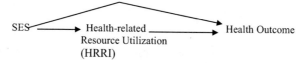

Using the same analytic strategy employed for relative deprivation, analyses are presented with reference to each of the component pathways between SES, resource utilization, and health outcomes (Figure 6.1) to determine whether these associations support the Fundamental Cause hypothesis. Given that the first component of the model, the association between SES and health outcomes, was clearly demonstrated in the previous chapter, the first phase of this analysis focuses on evaluating a new measure, the Health-Related Resource Index (HRRI).

Drawing on the idea that resource utilization reflects the propensity to use health-related resources in an effort to reduce risk and promote health, the HRRI reflects the frequency of engaging in selected health-promoting strategies. The HRRI was constructed as a summative index of health-promoting strategies that assigns an equal weight for each specific item. As such, an assumption was made that each resource item contributes equally to the profile of a health-related resource user (Rindskopf 1984). The conceptualization underlying the HRRI was not in the predictive value of its specific items, but rather in its ability to predict the universe of risk reduction strategies. Given the underlying assumptions of the HRRI, tests are conducted to assess 1) the predictive ability of the HRRI to capture the tendency to employ risk reduction strategies, and 2) whether the HRRI, which assumes equality of effect for each item, does not significantly differ from its individual components. To support the use of the HRRI, its predictive ability was assessed by posing the following question:

Is there evidence to suggest that the HRRI could predict the universe of health-related resource items?

As you may recall, the HRRI includes gender-specific health-related resources, thus, separate indexes are constructed for women and men. For women, the HRRI items include being physically active, not obese, not smoking, having health insurance, a flu shot, cholesterol screening, mammogram, breast exam, and a pap smear. The male HRRI was composed of being physically active, not obese, not smoking, having health insurance, a flu shot, cholesterol screening, and prostate screening.

To determine the HRRI's ability to predict this larger universe of health-related resources, indexes of all but one resource item are constructed to predict the likelihood of engaging in the remaining item. For example, if an index of eight items can predict the 9th remaining item, then potentially it can capture the 10th, 11th, etc. Figure 6.3 illustrates one example of this in the association between the frequencies of employing the six remaining self-care strategies in relation to the 7th resource item, non-smoking status. The proportion of male non-smokers increases in lock step as the frequency of employing health-promoting activities increases, suggesting that the index could predict a larger collection of health related resources.

Figure 6.3   Health-related Resources & Non-Smoking Status,
HRS Male Respondents, w3, n=4,385

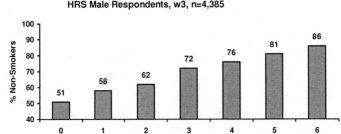

Similar patterns emerge among women. For example, Figure 6.4 illustrates that as the number of health-related resources increases, the percentage of female non-smokers increases, suggesting that engaging in a collection of health-promoting strategies may predict engaging in a whole host of health-promoting activities.

Figure 6.4   Health-related Resources & Non-Smoking Status,
                HRS Female Respondents, w3, n=5,402

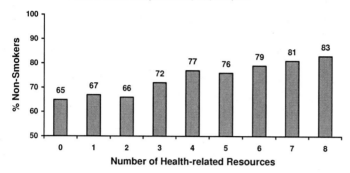

Identical analyses are conducted for all the selected resource items, and similar patterns to those illustrated above are found for both women and men (results not shown). Trends suggest that a collection of strategies predicts the remaining item, and ideally, captures the universe of health-promoting strategies.

Although the HRRI is predominantly comprised of health-promoting behavioral elements, health-related resource utilization differs from behavioral models in its conceptualization. Health behavior models typically indicate that SES causes the disadvantaged to engage in risk-related behavior at increased levels, which in turn, causes premature morbidity and mortality. Instead of examining behavior among the disadvantaged, Link and Phelan's Resource Utilization theory directs the focus to behavior as one proceeds up the hierarchy. As resources increase, one's ability to reduce risk-related behavior increases. Consequently, resource utilization generates the persistent association of risk-related behavior among the less advantaged as a function of being deprived of resources. As research uncovers mechanisms to reduce disability and death, those that are more advantaged can leverage resources to improve their health and longevity. While the methods to test these perspectives are essentially the same, the conceptualization and meaning of resource utilization and behavioral explanations differ. The measurement model for the HRRI is akin to one that might be constructed for a stressful life events scale. Stressful life event items are discrete occurrences such as job loss, death of a

78

spouse, or assault that are not conceptualized as emerging from a unitary underlying process. However, experiencing several events increases one's risk of psychiatric symptoms over experiencing none. Similarly, it was proposed that increased access to health-related resources should increase the likelihood of better health and longevity. To assess reliability for this type of scale, the test-retest method is recommended over internal consistency. Unfortunately, this method could not be conducted in the case of the HRRI since additional data necessary to conduct this method are not available.

Although the resource utilization process was not considered a latent construct, Cronbach's alpha was calculated nevertheless, and was found to be .47 for the female HRRI, and .42 for the male HRRI. As expected, the relatively modest degree of correlation between items confirms that the process as conceptualized doesn't actually fit a latent construct model, and indicates that the resource utilization scale is better conceptualized as factors that, when added together, reflect access to and utilization of health-related resources.

Given that empirical evidence suggests sufficient predictive ability of the HRRI, the next step to lend support for using this measure was to determine the utility of using the index as compared to its individual items as posed in the following question:

Do the estimation models, which contain the HRRI, differ significantly from those models that include the individual items?

To assess whether each indicator item contributes equally or whether some are more important than others, two sets of regression models are specified to predict SES indicators and health outcomes. Each set contains models that include the HRRI (Index Model) as compared to models using the individual components of the HRRI (Items Model). The Index models, which constrain each of the resource items to have an equal effect, for women and men, include the following:

SES Indicators (Income, Education, Net Worth) / Logit (Poor Health Outcome) = $b0 + b1_{HRRI} + b2_{race/ethnicity} + b11_{age} + b12_{marital\ status} + \varepsilon$

79

The full Items Model for women, which allows each item to have its own effect, includes the following:

SES Indicators (Income, Education, Net Worth) / Logit (Poor Health Outcome) = b0 + b1 $_{\text{physically active}}$ + b2 $_{\text{not obese}}$ + b3 $_{\text{non-smoker}}$ + b4 $_{\text{health insurance}}$ + b5 $_{\text{flu shot}}$ + b6 $_{\text{cholesterol screen}}$ + b7 $_{\text{mammogram}}$ + b8 $_{\text{breast exam}}$ + b9 $_{\text{pap smear}}$ + b10 $_{\text{race/ethnicity}}$ + b11 $_{\text{age}}$ + b12 $_{\text{marital status}}$ + ε

The full Items Model for men includes the following:

SES Indicators (Income, Education, Net Worth) / Logit (Poor Health Outcome) = b0 + b1 $_{\text{physically active}}$ + b2 $_{\text{not obese}}$ + b3 $_{\text{non-smoker}}$ + b4 $_{\text{health insurance}}$ + b5 $_{\text{flu shot}}$ + b6 $_{\text{cholesterol screen}}$ + b7 $_{\text{prostate screen}}$ + b8 $_{\text{race/ethnicity}}$ + b9 $_{\text{age}}$ + b10 $_{\text{marital status}}$ + ε

Models are compared using the following formula:

$$\frac{(R^2_2 - R^2_1) / J\text{-}1}{(1 - R^2_2) / N - (J\text{-}1)}$$

This equation was used to test whether a model with one group of parameters is significantly different than another model reflecting a different group of parameters (Judd and McClelland 1989). In this case, do models including the HRRI significantly differ from those that contain the individual items? The values for the above formula include R^2_2, which represents the r-square of the Items Model, R^2_1 represents the r-square of the Index Model, J-1 was calculated as the number of parameters estimated in the Items Model minus the number of parameters estimated in the Index Model (the degrees of freedom), and N represents the number of the strata within the sampling specifications.

Table 6.1 presents a detailed list of model comparison calculations stratified by gender and outcome measure. The second column of Table 6.1 represents the proportional reduction in error (PRE) which represents the proportion of error reduced between the Index model and the Items model. Essentially, the PRE represents the change in R-square between the models. The smaller the value of PRE, the more worthwhile it is to choose the simpler, more parsimonious model.

Calculating the F-value serves to examine the proportional reduction in error per additional parameter added to the model, and to compare the proportion of error that was reduced (PRE) to the proportion of error that remains (Judd and McClelland 1989). For the more

80

complex model to be considered to be a better fit in terms of reducing error rather than the simpler one, the F-value must exceed the critical F value based on the degrees of freedom or number of parameters estimated within each model. Calculations for both PRE and the F-value do not exceed their respective critical values. Hence, the more parsimonious Health-related Resource Index model was selected for all subsequent analyses.

Table 6.1 Health-related Resource Utilization Regression Model Comparison; (Limited to those with excellent/good health or having no conditions at W3)			
Resources →SES	Proportional Reduction in Error (PRE)	F-value	H_0: Models are not significantly different Reject H_0?
Women[1] (n=4,289)			
Household Income	.027	.150	No
Education	.023	.132	No
Household Net Worth	.016	.092	No
Men[2] (n=3,485)			
Household Income	.019	.128	No
Education	.028	.188	No
Household Net Worth	.014	.096	No
Resources →Health Outcomes	Women[1]		
Self-reported Health (n=4,289)	.050	.292	No
Having Any Conditions (n=3,670)	.024	.136	No
Mortality(n=5,902)	.006	.033	No
	Men[2]		
Self-reported Health (n=3,485)	.034	.196	No
Having Any Conditions (n=2,705)	.020	.156	No
Mortality (n=4,904)	.023	.184	No
Linear Regression used for outcomes: SES Indicators (Household Income, Education, and Household Net Worth) [1]$F_{(8, 40)}$ critical value ($\forall$=.05): 2.18; [2]$F_{(6, 40)}$ critical value ($\forall$=.05): 2.34 Logistic Regression used for outcomes: SRH, Conditions, and Mortality			

Using the HRRI, the analysis proceeds to examine each of the bivariate associations between SES, health-related resource utilization, and health outcomes. Some associations are depicted graphically to serve as illustrative examples, while the remaining associations are discussed in the text. The first component in the proposed causal chain prompts the following question:

Is SES associated with health-related resource utilization?

Figure 6.5 SES-Resource Utilization Model

SES ⟶ Resource Utilization

Although SES indicators and the HRRI are measured continuously for the multivariable analyses, these measures are categorized to demonstrate bivariate associations for illustrative purposes. Cut points for the HRRI categories are set to reflect a fairly equal distribution between categories. The top category of the female HRRI, employing 7 to 9 resources, reflects approximately one-third (37%) of the female respondents. Similarly, close to one-third (32%) of the respondents fall into the highest category of the male HRRI, which represents men who employ 6 to 7 resources. Chi-square tests indicate that household income (χ^2=26.6, df: 6, p<.001), household net worth (χ^2=22.2, df: 6, p<.001), and educational attainment (χ^2=15.5, df: 6, p<.001) significantly and positively influence resource utilization among women.

Figure 6.6   Household Income and Health-related Resource Utilization, HRS Female Respondents, W3, n=4,289

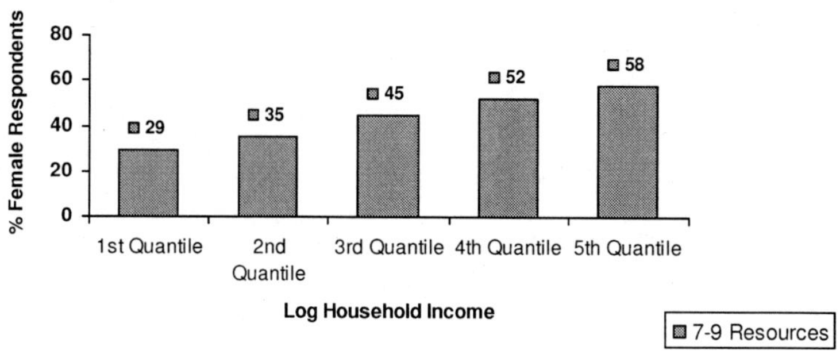

For example, Figure 6.6 illustrates the distribution of health-related resource utilization in relation to household income. As one compares the lowest (1st quantile) to the highest category of household income, proportions of women who employ 7 to 9 health-related resources increases.

A similar pattern emerges among men with respect to SES indicators and resource utilization. Chi-square tests indicate that increasing levels of resource utilization are clearly associated with increasing levels of household income (χ^2=18.4, df: 6, p<.001), education (χ^2=14, df: 6, p<.001), and household net worth (χ^2=16, df: 6, p<.001) among men. For example, Figure 6.7 clearly illustrates that increasing household income shapes the extent to which men engage in the highest number of health-related resources.

82

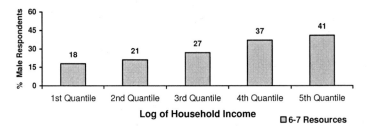

Figure 6.7   Household Income and Health-related Resource Utilization, HRS Male Respondents, W3-W4, n=3,485

Bivariate tests demonstrate that increasing absolute resources, as specified by the three SES indicators, was significantly predictive of employing health-related resources to reduce health risks and promote health among women and men. The next component in the causal model to be examined prompts the following inquiry:

Is health-related resource utilization associated with health outcomes?

Figure 6.8 Health-related Resource Utilization-Health Outcomes Model

Health-related Resource Utilization ⟶ Health Outcomes

To examine the relationship between health-related resource utilization and health outcomes, chi-square tests are conducted for each of the three health outcome variables. Tests indicate that the lower the number of resources employed, the higher the proportion of women experience poor self-reported health status (χ^2=30, df: 2, p<.001), having any life-threatening conditions (χ^2=21, df: 2, p<.01), and death (χ^2=20, df: 2, p<.001) as illustrated in Figure 6.9. For men, a slightly different pattern emerges between health-related resource utilization and health outcomes.

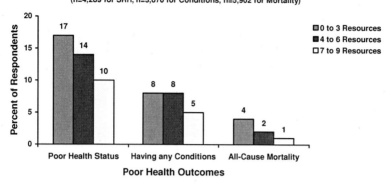

Figure 6.9   Health-related Resource Utilization & Poor Health
Outcomes, HRS Female Respondents, W3-W4,
(n=4,289 for SRH, n=3,670 for Conditions, n=5,902 for Mortality)

As illustrated in Figure 6.10, bivariate chi-square tests indicate that higher proportions of poor self-rated health (χ^2=23, df: 2, p<.001) are inversely and significantly associated with lower levels of health-related resource utilization, while resource utilization was not found to significantly influence having any life-threatening conditions (χ^2=6, df: 2, p=.30) or mortality (χ^2=4, df: 2, p=.20) among men.

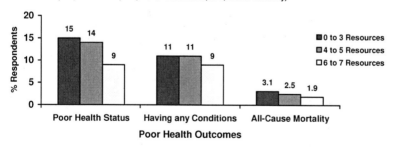

Figure 6.10   Health-related Resource Utilization & Poor Health
Outcomes, HRS Male Respondents, W3-W4,
(n=3,485 for SRH, n=2,705 for Conditions, n=4,904 for Mortality)

While bivariate results indicate that SES was firmly linked to resource utilization among men and women, the association between resource utilization and health outcomes is less clear. Although low resource utilization was significantly associated with all poor health outcomes among women, low resource utilization was significantly associated with poor health status only among men. To confirm these findings, component pathways are re-examined in the following analyses using regression techniques within a multivariable context, and the HRRI was modified back to a continuous, rather than a categorical, measure to utilize the full extent of resource utilization data. The next component of the causal chain prompts the following question:

Is health-related resource utilization predictive of health status, morbidity and mortality, controlling for SES?

Figure 6.11 SES-Resource utilization-Health Outcomes Model

SES ⟶ Health–related ⟶ Health Outcomes
Resource
Utilization

Similar to the analytic strategy used in the Relative Deprivation analyses, multivariable models are developed to test two hypotheses concerning the components of the causal chain depicted in Figure 6.11. Specifically, analyses explore whether SES is predictive of resource utilization, adjusting for demographic covariates. Models are also estimated to determine whether resource utilization mediates the association between SES and health outcomes.

Hypothesis Testing

The first hypothesis indicates that increasing socioeconomic status will be associated with health-related resource utilization, and will not differ in terms of age, race/ethnicity, and marital status. Table 6.2 presents estimates of the linear regression models examining the discrete SES components underlying this assumption for both men and women.

Models 1 through 4 confirm bivariate associations within a multivariable context such that increasing household income (b= .165, p<.001), educational attainment (b=.095, p<.001), and household net worth (b= .398, p<.01) are significantly predictive of increasing health-related resource utilization among women. Similar patterns are found among men (household income: b= .121, p<.001, educational attainment: b=.077, p<.001, and household net worth: b= .304, p<.001). A set of covariates was added in model 5 to control for potential confounding in the effect of SES on health-related resource utilization. In the full model, SES indicators remain significantly associated with resource utilization in the expected direction.

Table 6.2	Health-related Resource Utilization Models; Limited to those with excellent/good health at W3								
	Women (n=4,289)					Men (n=4,305)				
Covariates	Model 1 Beta (SE)	Model 2 Beta (SE)	Model 3 Beta (SE)	Model 4 Beta (SE)	Model 5 Beta (SE)	Model 1 Beta (SE)	Model 2 Beta (SE)	Model 3 Beta (SE)	Model 4 Beta (SE)	Model 5 Beta (SE)
Log Household Income	.248† (.020)			.165† (.018)	.128† (.018)	.208† (.023)			.121† (.022)	.104† (.021)
Education		.145† (.012)		.095† (.012)	.102† (.012)		.108† (.009)		.077† (.009)	.083† (.010)
Log Household Net Worth			.803† (.110)	.398** (.110)	.300** (.108)			.612† (.059)	.304† (.052)	.252† (.051)
Race/ Ethnicity										
White[a]					.060 (.088)					.029 (.098)
Hispanic[a]					-.176 (.200)					-.058 (.135)
Other[a]					-.032 (.239)					-.262 (.253)
Age					.012 (.010)					.037† (.008)
Married[b]					.407† (.083)					.443† (.082)
R^2	.05	.04	.03	.07	.08	.05	.04	.03	.07	.09

Linear Regression used for outcome: Health-related Resource Utilization
[a] Compared to Blacks;
[b] Compared to never married, divorced, widowed, or separated   *p<.05, **p<.01, †p<.001

In terms of demographic covariates, being married or living with a partner as compared to those who are unmarried, was significantly predictive of increasing resource utilization, adjusting for SES and other covariates among women and men. Increasing age persists as a significant predictor of resource utilization as well as being married among men only. Findings suggest that cohabitation, or some component within its context, was significantly associated with increasing resource utilization for men and women, across SES levels. In terms of age and resource utilization among men, higher resource utilization may be related to aging as a function of being engaged in the health care system, particularly for prostate screening and cholesterol screening. In contrast, women are more likely to be engaged in the care system throughout their adult lives, particularly with respect to gynecological services, and thus, resource utilization would not significantly differ by age. Although increasing SES persists as significantly predictive of increasing resource utilization within a multivariable context among men and women, results also indicate that resource utilization differs by marital status for women, and by age and marital status for men. As such, results provide some support for the first hypothesis.

The second hypothesis postulates that health-related resource utilization will mediate the SES–health association. To mediate this association, the size of the direct effect of SES on the outcome variables should be substantially reduced and the mediator should remain significantly predictive in the expected direction within the full model. For each of the three outcome variables, a sequence of logistic regression equations was estimated. The baseline model, model 1, estimates the direct effect of each SES indicator on the outcome variable. The second model adds a set of demographic covariates including race/ethnicity, age and marital status to control for possible spurious effects that may confound the SES-health outcome association. The third model measures the direct effect of health-related resource utilization on a health outcome, and the fourth model examines the effect of health-related resource utilization, adjusting for demographic covariates. The final model includes the SES indicators, health-related resource utilization, and demographic covariates to examine whether health-related resource utilization acts as a mediator. The equation for the full model was as follows:

$$\text{Logit (Poor Health Outcome)} = b1_{\text{income}} + b2_{\text{education}} + b3_{\text{net worth}} + b4_{\text{resource utilization}} + b5_{\text{race/ethnicity}} + b6_{\text{age}} + b7_{\text{marital status}} + \varepsilon$$

The first three terms on the right hand side of this equation controls for household income, net worth, and educational attainment. It was expected that the coefficient for these three terms demonstrate an inverse relationship with poor health outcomes. That is, the wealthier and wiser will be healthier. The fourth term represents the frequency of employing health-promoting strategies. As indicated in the previous chapter, the coefficient for this term should be significantly associated with the health outcome in the expected direction while the coefficients for the SES indicators should be reduced when the resource utilization term is added into the model for resource utilization to be considered a mediator. Logistic regression coefficients for the SES variables are compared across models to assess the effect of resource utilization. To aid the reader in interpreting the effect of variables on the log odds of an outcome measure, adjusted odds ratios are reported for a specific set of values for the SES predictors.

Self-Rated Health Status

Table 6.3 examines the underlying assumption that health-related resource utilization is related to poor health status, controlling for SES, among women. It presents logistic regression coefficients for the effect of SES and resource utilization measured at wave 3 to predict health outcomes at wave 4, with and without adjustment for demographic characteristics.

Table 6.3 Poor Self-Rated Health Status Coefficients from Explanatory Models (W3-W4; Limited to those with excellent/good health at W3)

WOMEN *(n=4,289)*

Covariates	Model 1 Beta (SE)	Model 2 Beta (SE)	Model 3 Beta (SE)	Model 4 Beta (SE)	Model 5 Beta (SE)
Log Household Income	-.076* (.028)	-.048 (.030)			-.046 (.031)
Education	-.171† (.024)	-.177† (.025)			-.175† (.025)
Log Household Net Worth	-.890** (.264)	-.654* (.262)			-.638* (.266)
Health-related Resource Utilization			-.121†	-.090** (.027)	-.024 (.030)
Race/ Ethnicity					
White [a]		-.458** (.126)		-.700† (.126)	-.458** (.126)
Hispanic [a]		-.320 (.240)		.124 (.222)	-.326 (.241)
Other [a]		-.948 (.519)		-1.140* (.553)	-.954 (.519)
Age		-.029 (.019)		-.015 (.020)	-.028 (.019)
Married [b]		-.340* (.132)		-.398** (.119)	-.332* (.131)

Logistic Regression used for outcome: Self-Rated Health
[a] Compared to Blacks;
[b] Compared to never married, divorced, widowed, or separated   *p<.05, **p<.01, † p<.001

Models 1 and 2 reflect the persistent and significant influence of decreasing SES on poor health status among women, particularly during a relatively short observation period (2 years). Household income (b= -.076, p<.05) educational attainment (b= -.171, p<.001) and household net worth (b= -.890, p<.01) are significantly and inversely associated with poor health status. Among women who reported good/excellent health status at wave 3, the odds of reporting poor self-rated health at wave 4 are 1.14 times larger for women in the 10th percentile of household income as compared to women within the 90th percentile, holding other SES indicators constant. Comparing women high school graduates to women who graduated college, the odds of reporting poor self-rated health are approximately doubled (1.9) for high school graduates. Models 3 and 4 indicate increasing health-related resource utilization (b= -.090, p<.01) persists as inversely and significantly associated with poor health status, with and without adjustment for covariates. Increasing resource utilization, on average, significantly reduces the odds of reporting poor health status (OR=.886, p<.001, CI: .838, .936). Simply, the odds of reporting poor self-reported health are close to two (1.82) times greater for women who report engaging in 2 health-related resources as compared to women who report engaging in 7 health-related resources.

When resource utilization was included with SES indicators and demographic covariates in model 5, resource utilization does not persist as a significant predictor among women. Furthermore, the addition of resource utilization does not substantially reduce the direct effect of any of the SES indicators. Hence, evidence does not support the hypothesis that resource utilization mediates the SES-health association among women. Being black and unmarried remains significantly predictive of poor health status across all models. Results echo other research findings (Williams 1999) which indicate that race conveys additional health disadvantage beyond that accounted for by SES.

Does health-related resource utilization operate in a similar fashion among men? Table 6.4 displays the estimates of logistic regression models to examine the role of health-related resource utilization among men. Similar to women, household net worth (b= -.528, p<.05) and educational attainment (b= -.122, p<.001) persist as significantly and inversely predictive of poor health status. What was different was that household income (b= -.102, p<.01) appears to have a stronger effect among men in its magnitude and persisting statistical significance across all models. While decreasing resource utilization was significantly associated with poor health status among men, even after adjustment for demographic covariates, it does not remain significantly associated with poor health status when SES indicators are included as shown in model 5. Comparing models 2 and 5, the addition of resource utilization does not substantially reduce the SES coefficients. As such, resource utilization does not appear to mediate the SES-health status association among men or women.

89

Table 6.4	Poor Self-Rated Health Status Coefficients from Explanatory Models (W3-W4) Limited to those with excellent/good health at W3				
	MEN *(n=3,485)*				
Covariates	*Model 1* Beta (SE)	*Model 2* Beta (SE)	*Model 3* Beta (SE)	*Model 4* Beta (SE)	*Model 5* Beta (SE)
Log Household Income	-.116** (.034)	-.102** (.032)			-.100** (.034)
Education	-.120† (.019)	-.122† (.024)			-.119† (.023)
Log Household Net Worth	-.592* (.234)	-.528* (.232)			-.516* (.229)
Health-related Resource Utilization			-.139† (.035)	-.112** (.036)	-.028 (.036)
Race/ Ethnicity					
White [a]		-.445* (.182)		-.784† (.169)	-.446* (.181)
Hispanic [a]		-.592* (.274)		-.238 (.223)	-.595* (.275)
Other [a]		-.442 (.410)		-.878* (.389)	-.456 (.403)
Age		-.001 (.021)		.013 (.020)	-.0003 (.021)
Married [b]		-.263 (.185)		-.292 (.186)	-.251 (.187)

Logistic Regression used for outcomes: Self-Rated Health
[a] Compared to Blacks;
[b] Compared to never married, divorced, widowed, or separated   *p<.05, **p<.01, †p<.001

Although being black persists as significantly predictive of poor health status, marriage was not found to significantly influence poor health status among men. The analysis proceeds to examine resource utilization in relation to SES and having any life-threatening conditions.

Having Any Life-threatening Conditions

The role of resource utilization in influencing the onset of life-threatening conditions with respect to SES among women is explored within Table 6.5. Recall that the sample was limited to women without any life-threatening conditions at wave 3 to predict the onset of conditions at wave 4. Models 1 and 2 indicate that decreasing household income (b= -.089, p<.01) and low educational attainment (b= -.083, p<.01) are significantly predictive of having any conditions life-threatening among women. The odds of having any conditions at wave 4 are 1.3 times greater for women in the 10th percentile of household income as compared to women within the 90th percentile, holding other SES indicators constant.

Table 6.5	Having Any Life-threatening Conditions Coefficients from Explanatory Models (W3-W4) Limited to those without any conditions at W3				
	WOMEN *(n=3,670)*				
Covariates	*Model 1* Beta (SE)	*Model 2* Beta (SE)	*Model 3* Beta (SE)	*Model 4* Beta (SE)	*Model 5* Beta (SE)
Log Household Income	-.100** (.036)	-.089* (.037)			-.083* (.038)
Education	-.065* (.028)	-.083* (.031)			-.076* (.032)
Log Household Net Worth	-.659* (.314)	-.625 (.325)			-.586 (.314)
Health-related Resource Utilization			-.131† (.035)	-.113** (.035)	-.058 (.036)
Race/ Ethnicity					
White [a]		.093 (.207)		-.116 (.201)	.087 (.208)
Hispanic [a]		-.285 (.330)		.093 (.306)	-.283 (.326)
Other [a]		.443 (.476)		.214 (.467)	.434 (.469)
Age		.028 (.021)		.032 (.022)	.029 (.021)
Married [b]		-.239 (.204)		-.371 (.202)	-.214 (.206)
Logistic Regression used for outcomes: Having Any Life-threatening Conditions [a] Compared to Blacks; [b] Compared to never married, divorced, widowed, or separated				*p<.05, **p<.01, †p<.001	

Women who completed high school are 30% more likely to report having any life-threatening conditions as compared to those women who completed college. In terms of household net worth, the odds for those women who reside in a household within the 10th percentile of the net worth distribution are 22% more likely to report having any conditions as compared to those women within the 90th percentile of household net worth.

Decreasing resource utilization (b= -.113, p<.01) was significantly associated with having any life-threatening conditions among women, with and without adjustment for demographic covariates as indicated in models 3 and 4. However, resource utilization does not remain significantly predictive of having any conditions when SES was controlled. When comparing models 2 and 5, the direct effect of SES indicators was not reduced when resource utilization was added into the full model. Findings indicate that although resource utilization was significantly related to both SES and having any conditions, it does not act to mediate the SES-conditions association among women.

Does resource utilization operate in a similar fashion in relation to having any conditions among men? Logistic regression results for men are presented in Table 6.6. What is most apparent from Table 6.6 is that none of the variables across all models are significantly associated with the onset of having any conditions. These results are particularly surprising in light of the robust and persistent association between SES and health outcomes. Though surprising, the lack of expected findings may reflect the relatively short observation period (2 years). If one were to examine the onset of conditions over a longer time period results may differ. However, this pattern is not reflected in the association between having any conditions and resource utilization among women.

Table 6.6 Having Any Life-threatening Conditions Coefficients from Explanatory Models (W3-W4) Limited to those without any conditions at W3

			MEN (n=2,705)		
Covariates	Model 1 Beta (SE)	Model 2 Beta (SE)	Model 3 Beta (SE)	Model 4 Beta (SE)	Model 5 Beta (SE)
Log Household Income	-.001 (.041)	.025 (.045)			.030 (.045)
Education	-.022 (.019)	-.009 (.021)			-.003 (.022)
Log Household Net Worth	-.082 (.134)	-.109 (.129)			-.094 (.131)
Health-related Resource Utilization			-.063 (.044)	-.057 (.044)	-.056 (.045)
Race/Ethnicity					
White [a]		-.213 (.218)		-.225 (.213)	-.215 (.219)
Hispanic [a]		.055 (.298)		.043 (.293)	.052 (.299)
Other [a]		-1.299 (.771)		-1.335 (.762)	-1.327 (.770)
Age		.045 (.025)		.046 (.025)	.048 (.025)
Married [b]		-.172 (.251)		-.125 (.240)	-.142 (.249)

Logistic Regression used for outcomes: Having Any Life-threatening Conditions
[a] Compared to Blacks;
[b] Compared to never married, divorced, widowed, or separated   *p<.05, **p<.01, †p<.001

Although it remains unclear as to why having any conditions as an outcome variable should yield such results, perhaps the mechanisms surrounding the onset of a life-threatening condition differ from poor health status and mortality. Nonetheless, resource utilization was examined in relation to the last health outcome, mortality.

All-Cause Mortality

Models examining the effects of SES and resource utilization on mortality between wave 3 and 4 among women are presented in Table 6.7. Models 1 and 2 indicate that household income (b= -.149, p<.001) and household net worth (b= -1.393, p<.01) are significantly predictive of mortality among women.

Table 6.7 Mortality Coefficients from Explanatory Models (W3-W4)					
Women (n=5,902)					
Covariates	*Model 1* Beta (SE)	*Model 2* Beta (SE)	*Model 3* Beta (SE)	*Model 4* Beta (SE)	*Model 5* Beta (SE)
Log Household Income	-.153† (.034)	-.149† (.034)			-.138† (.033)
Education	.003 (.035)	.019 (.034)			.036 (.036)
Log Household Net Worth	-1.361* (.526)	-1.393* (.577)			-1.222* (.586)
Health-related Resource Utilization			-.242† (.051)	-.222† (.055)	-.184** (.057)
Race/ Ethnicity					
White [a]		-.195 (.227)		-.446 (.232)	-.235 (.233)
Hispanic [a]		.028 (.354)		.075 (.353)	.014 (.350)
Other [a]		-.399 (1.035)		-.638 (1.036)	-.410 (1.044)
Age		.061 (.039)		.060 (.039)	.065 (.039)
Married [b]		.021 (.213)		-.272 (.213)	.083 (.220)
Logistic Regression used for outcomes: All-Cause Mortality [a] Compared to Blacks; [b] Compared to never married, divorced, widowed, or separated †p<.001				*p<.05, **p<.01,	

All other factors being equal, the odds of women in the 10th percentile of household income are 1.5 times greater than those women within the 90th percentile. Similarly, the odds of women in the 10th percentile of household net worth are twice that of those women within the 90th percentile. However, within the multivariable context, educational attainment was not significantly associated with mortality, nor was it found to be associated in the expected direction as shown in models 1 and 2. Results suggest that collinearity between the SES indicators may be operating to alter the sign of the educational attainment coefficient as a result of the strong direct effect of household income and net worth. Models 3 and 4 reveal that increasing resource utilization (b= -.222, p<.001) among women significantly influences mortality, with and without adjustment for demographic characteristics. For example, the odds of dying are 30% greater for women who report engaging in 2 health-related resources as compared to women who report engaging in 7 health-related resources.

Increasing resource utilization persists as significantly predictive of mortality among women, controlling for SES, as indicated in the full model (model 5). To assess whether resource utilization mediates the SES-mortality association, models 2 and 5 are compared. Findings indicate that the direct effect of household net worth was reduced by 12%. As such, health-related resource utilization may be mediating some portion of the relationship between SES and mortality among women.

The association between SES, resource utilization, and mortality was examined among men as presented in Table 6.8. Similar to the findings among women, models 1 and 2 indicate that decreasing household income (b= -.099, p<.01) and household net worth (b=-1.380, p<.01) are significantly predictive of mortality. Although educational attainment does not reach statistical significance, its association to mortality was found to occur in the expected direction. That is, lower educational attainment was associated with mortality. Among men, increasing age and being black as compared to Hispanic, are associated with mortality across all models. Health-related resource utilization (b=-.191, p<.01) persists as significantly predictive of mortality among men, with and without adjustment for covariates. For example, the odds of dying are 1.8 times greater for men who report engaging in 2 health-related resources as compared to men who report engaging in 6 health-related resources.

Table 6.8 Mortality Coefficients from Explanatory Models (W3-W4)

Covariates	Model 1 Beta (SE)	Model 2 Beta (SE)	Model 3 Beta (SE)	Model 4 Beta (SE)	Model 5 Beta (SE)
	Men (n=4,904)				
Log Household Income	-.081** (.027)	-.099** (.029)			-.089** (.032)
Education	-.022 (.031)	-.022 (.035)			-.012 (.036)
Log Household Net Worth	-1.225** (.444)	-1.380** (.468)			-1.313** (.469)
Health-related Resource Utilization			-.164** (.053)	-.191** (.054)	-.129* (.062)
Race/ Ethnicity					
White [a]		-.311 (.277)		-.541 (.279)	-.300 (.279)
Hispanic [a]		-1.206** (.537)		-1.095* (.526)	-1.218* (.539)
Other [a]		-.924 (.814)		-1.222 (.845)	-.997 (.825)
Age		.097** (.034)		.101** (.034)	.102** (.034)
Married [b]		.418 (.307)		.258 (.293)	.467 (.311)

Logistic Regression used for outcomes: Having Any Life-threatening Conditions
[a] Compared to Blacks;
[b] Compared to never married, divorced, widowed, or separated   *p<.05, **p<.01, †p<.001

With respect to assessing mediation, health-related resource utilization remains statistically predictive of mortality in the correct direction when comparing models 2 and 5. In addition, the direct effect of household income was reduced (10%) when resource utilization was added into the model. Results suggest that resource utilization may be mediating a small portion of the SES-mortality association.

Summary of Findings

While increasing SES was significantly predictive of increasing health resource utilization among men and women, the association between increasing health-related resource utilization and better health outcomes is less clear. Table 6.9 presents a summary of the findings in relation to health-related resource utilization across health outcomes for women and men.

Table 6.9 Summary of Health-related Resource Utilization Findings

Multivariable Regression Models		WOMEN	MEN
SES→ Health-related Resource Utilization		**Positively associated?**	
	Household Income	Yes	Yes
	Education	Yes	Yes
	Household Net Worth	Yes	Yes
Health-related Resource Utilization→ Better Health Outcomes		**Positively associated?**	
	SRH	Yes	Yes
	Conditions	Yes	No
	Mortality	Yes	Yes
SES→ Health-related Resource Utilization → Better Health Outcomes		Does Mediation Occur?	
	SES→Health-related Resource Utilization→SRH	No	No
	SES→ Health-related Resource Utilization→Conditions	No	No
	SES→ Health-related Resource Utilization→Mortality	Yes	Yes

The first component in the proposed causal chain derived from the Fundamental Cause perspective posits that SES will be positively predictive of health-related resource utilization. Results confirm this claim in that increasing SES was significantly associated with increasing health-related resource utilization. The second hypothesis indicates that health-related resource utilization will be positively associated with improved health outcomes. Although resource utilization was not found to be associated with having any life-threatening conditions among men, the remaining five tests indicate a statistically significant association in the expected direction, suggesting that health-related resource utilization is associated to a large extent to improved health outcomes. These findings are consistent with Link and Phelan's description of how SES facilitates an individual to engage in healthy behaviors and avail themselves of the newest technological innovations, as well as how health-promoting strategies influence health outcomes.

While findings indicate that the component pathways of the proposed causal chain operate as theorized in that SES was predictive of health-related resource utilization, and in general, health-related resource utilization was predictive of improved health outcomes, results also indicate that health-related resource utilization as measured does not account for the SES-health association in the case of self-reported health status and having any life-threatening conditions.

Although resource utilization was found to mediate some portion of the SES-mortality association for both women and men, the effect was very modest. Despite the modest effect, inconsistent findings prompted further analysis to determine whether the effect of health-related resource utilization on mortality influences survival once an individual was ill or had been diagnosed with a life-threatening condition, rather than delaying the onset of life-threatening illness or disability. Two variables were developed to reflect: 1) the interaction between resource utilization and having any conditions, and 2) the interaction between resource utilization and poor health status. Estimation models were specified to include these interaction variables to predict mortality. Interactions were not found to be significantly associated with mortality for women and men (results not shown).

In general, empirical evidence does not suggest that resource utilization as specified accounts for, or explains the SES-health association. Thus, it does not appear to serve as a primary mechanism through which SES influences health outcomes. Further discussion and implications of the findings are discussed in the final chapter.

Chapter VII

An Assessment of the Evidence and its Implications

In the debate concerning SES disparities in health, is relative deprivation or resource utilization driving the SES-health gradient within industrialized societies? This study sought to examine the contribution of psychosocial processes as described in Wilkinson's theory of relative deprivation, as compared to materialist factors as described in Link and Phelan's Fundamental Cause explanation, to account for the association between SES and health outcomes. The following discussion summarizes the results, and outlines the implications of the findings with reference to further research and public policy.

Overall summary of findings

The theoretical perspective proposed by Wilkinson (1985) indicates that relative deprivation, a social comparison process which engenders perceptions of economic deprivation relative to a reference group, adversely affects health within industrialized societies. If this theory is operating as described, what empirical findings would one expect to find? One might expect to find that those at the top of a low-income group should experience better health outcomes as compared to those at the bottom of a high-income group, absolute income level being approximately equal.

To test this premise, efforts were made to identify a situation where the two conditions of the theory would be met such that individuals would differ with respect to relative income while absolute income would be similar. By carving out a portion of the sample limited to the top and bottom 10% of the zip code income distribution, respondents could be categorized by absolute and relative income into four subgroups: the bottom of the high-income group, the top of the high-income group, the bottom of the low-income group, and the top of the low-income group. According to Wilkinson, relative deprivation would predict that those at the bottom of a high-income group would perceive themselves to be economically deprived relative to those around them, and thus, reflect a higher prevalence of poor health outcomes. However, actual proportions of health outcomes were found to indicate the opposite. Prevalence of poor health outcomes were greater for those at top of the low-income group as compared to those respondents who fell into the bottom of a high-income group, although the average income levels of these subgroups were similar. While this strategic comparison test leaves out a significant portion of data by only including 20% of the sample, it reflects the extremes of the income distribution. As such, one would expect to find the effects of relative deprivation among these groups, if anywhere, for it to be operating as Wilkinson has suggested. The results of this strategic comparison test did not support Wilkinson's hypothesis.

Statistical models were developed to further investigate the role of relative income and financial dissatisfaction within a multivariable context. The direct effect of SES on health outcomes was examined as compared with those models that included relative income and financial dissatisfaction, with and without adjustment for demographic covariates. Regression analyses of the pathways between SES and relative income clearly indicated that increasing SES is positively associated with relative income. While relative income tends to fail as a predictor within the full multivariable models, low relative income is found to significantly predict financial dissatisfaction for men and women, adjusting for SES, although the association was weaker for women. In addition, low relative income was found to be significantly predictive of all three health outcomes, adjusting for covariates, among women and men in the expected direction.

Findings further support Wilkinson's hypothesis in that financial dissatisfaction is found to reduce SES effects, and persist as a significant predictor of health outcomes at or below the .05 significance level in four of the six tests for mediation.

In comparison to the Relative Deprivation perspective, Fundamental Cause theory emphasizes the utilization of resources to promote health and reduce risk as the mechanism underlying the persistence of the SES-health gradient. To explore this claim, multivariable regression models were developed to assess whether the extent to which one employs or engages in health-promoting or risk-reduction resources partially accounts for the SES-health relationship. Gender-specific resource utilization scales were constructed to measure the extent of resource utilization. Tests were found to suggest that the scales included sufficient predictive ability and parsimony in relation to resource utilization.

Increasing SES as well as better health outcomes were found to be independently and significantly linked to increasing health-related resource utilization. In particular, increasing household income, education and net worth increases the odds of utilizing an increasing number of health-related resources. Similarly, increasing resource utilization is significantly predictive of better health and survival. However, for two of the three health outcomes tested, resource utilization did not strongly mediate the SES-health association. In the case of the third outcome, mortality, the effect of resource utilization is fairly small. Findings indicate that health-related resource utilization as measured does not explain, or account for, the SES-health gradient. Before an interpretation of the findings is provided, potential limitations of the study are considered.

Limitations

Several limitations of the study are important to consider with reference to the findings and their relationship to the theoretical frameworks. First, analyzing longitudinal national data to answer questions not originally posed presents challenges in that available measures, though sufficient, are not ideal. For example, the financial dissatisfaction variable reflects responses to the question of whether one is dissatisfied with one's financial situation, but does not refer to any comparison process or a reference group. Thus, financial dissatisfaction also may reflect frustration with actually making ends meet, regardless of income level. While models indicate that decreasing relative income position is significantly predictive of increasing financial dissatisfaction, controlling for SES, the ability to conclude that financial dissatisfaction solely derives from relative income position is limited.

A second limitation is closely related to the first. The health-related resource index (HRRI) is very limited in summarizing the universe of health-promoting and risk-reducing strategies that individuals might engage in. It is probable that additional strategies not studied explain more of the relationship between SES and health outcomes. Some important health-related resources such as specific dietary habits, safe occupational environment, health-promoting leisure activity, resource-rich neighborhood, seat belt use, and other health-relevant circumstances were not included in the HRS dataset. Thus, only a subset of health-related resources was investigated. Moreover, using measures collected at one point in time does not fully capture the impact of resources over the life course, and thus, its effect on health and longevity. Nonetheless, the set of health-related resources used are directly related to reducing the major causes of morbidity and mortality such as heart disease and cancer (U.S. Department of Health and Human Services 2000).

Thirdly, the length of the follow-up period in the resource utilization analyses (2 years) is relatively short, limiting the extent to which one can explore the longer term effects of SES with respect to resource utilization on health outcomes. Preventive health resource items such as cholesterol screening were not collected until 1996 during the third wave of the HRS. These limitations highlight the need for a study that is designed and implemented with the main purpose of testing the relative importance of relative deprivation versus resource utilization as explanations for SES gradients in health.

The fourth limitation is concerned with the operationalization of the reference group. This study used three different geographic aggregations, the zip code, county and state, to define its reference standard with regard to social comparison processes. Although geographic aggregations are typically used in studies of inequality and health, this measure assumes that people compare their income to incomes of those in relative proximity to themselves. However, people may also compare themselves in terms of income to the incomes of those within their occupational group, within their age range, among those with similar education, and within other demographic groups, regardless of geographic boundary. In addition, income comparison processes may occur with respect to oneself at an earlier time in life. Consequently, this comparison standard may be limited in detecting the full effect of relative deprivation. Limitations also include a potential bias which may result from limiting the prospective cohorts to those who reported excellent/good self-reported health and not having any life-threatening conditions. By limiting on these outcome measures, the effects of SES on health outcomes may be attenuated as a result of eliminating those respondents who have already fallen prey to the process. On the other hand, if this bias was significant, the association between SES and health would have disappeared. However, the robust association between SES and health outcomes persisted, even after those with poor health and any life-threatening conditions were excluded Lastly, the HRS survey sample was chosen as a data source because of its rich array of financial information, coupled with an extensive section on health status and behavior. It was designed to examine how socioeconomic status relates to quality of life and retirement during middle and early old age. As a result, the survey is limited to respondents within the 51-61 year old age range in 1992. As such, findings can be generalized to individuals considered to be in late middle age or early old age.

Research has demonstrated that as one ages, financial dissatisfaction is shown to decrease (Schieman 2001). Others have found relative deprivation effects to be weaker among those 65 and older (Eibner and Evans 2001). Thus, this sample may be limited in estimating the extent of relative deprivation effects on health.

Interpretation of Findings

Findings from the relative deprivation analysis provide some evidence to support Wilkinson's hypothesis. Increasing SES is predictive of increasing relative income. Not surprising, since individuals with high income levels typically reside in affluent residential areas, causing income and relative income to be highly correlated. More importantly, decreasing relative income is predictive of financial dissatisfaction, regardless of absolute income level, indicating that income position is related to negative psychosocial mechanisms throughout the social hierarchy as suggested by Wilkinson. Furthermore, financial dissatisfaction was found to persist as significantly predictive of poor health and mortality, holding SES constant, for women and men. These findings are consistent with Wilkinson's claim that relative income position generates negative psychosocial consequences such as financial dissatisfaction, which in turn, increase the risk of poor health outcomes and mortality.

On the other hand, while evidence is consistent with Wilkinson's hypothesis as indicated above, relative income did not persist as significantly predictive of health outcomes within the full model. Thus, the role of relative deprivation as a mediator in the SES-health association was not supported. The sign of the coefficient of relative income was found to change to a positive value within the full model in five of the six tests conducted which is the opposite sign from that predicted by Wilkinson. Relative income, household income and median zip code income are found to be collinear, which means two of these variables perfectly predicts the third. Additional analyses not shown indicate that if one replicates the analyses using median income, rather than income difference, similar results are found. The strategic comparison tests and the full regression models indicate that better health outcomes are experienced by those at the bottom of the income ladder within a high-income area, as compared to those at the top of a lower-income area. Results suggest that relative deprivation is operating, but that the effect is not strong enough so as to produce the overall effect that Wilkinson suggests. Otherwise, the effect of relative income would have been observed, particularly with regard to the strategic comparison test where the effects are presumed to be the strongest.

Overall then, while findings are consistent with the possibility that relative deprivation influences health outcomes, it is clear that other mechanisms also influence health outcomes. In contrast to Wilkinson's hypothesis, results suggest that living within a high-income neighborhood may convey some contextual health-protective effect, regardless of individual income. These findings are consistent with the findings from the strategic comparison test which, again, contradicts Wilkinson's hypothesis. Findings are also consistent with the work of Diez-Roux and colleagues in that living in an advantaged neighborhood is found to significantly reduce the incidence of heart disease, even after adjusting for individual SES (Diez-Roux et al. 2001). If there is some contextual health-protective effect, what might be generating it? Some have suggested that these contextual effects may reflect the level and quality of public resources available in high-income communities, as well as the prevalence of health-promoting behavioral norms that influence health-related behavior (Lynch 2000).

Although the analyses do not allow us to definitively separate out the effects of relative income from other factors, findings suggest that relative deprivation is operating, although the effect is not as strong as Wilkinson has suggested. As such, relative deprivation is not considered the primary mechanism through which SES shapes health outcomes.

Evidence is found to support Wilkinson's hypothesis in that position within the social hierarchy is related to negative psychosocial consequences such as financial dissatisfaction, which in turn, negatively affects health. Though the mediating effects are modest, psychosocial mechanisms related to SES are found to be significantly associated with health outcomes. Findings suggest that the psychosocial burden of discontent as measured by financial dissatisfaction is operating throughout the social spectrum to effect health. In some sense, "keeping up with the joneses'" may be one of the factors acting to increase one's risk of morbidity and mortality.

While some of the findings of this study support Wilkinson's hypothesis, other population health patterns challenge the theory. If lower hierarchical position causes stress, which in turn, negatively affects health outcomes, SES would be consistently associated with stress-related conditions over time (Link and Phelan 2000). However, the changing patterns of risk for disease in relation to SES stand in stark contrast to this assertion. For decades, higher SES has been consistently associated with breast cancer mortality. More recently, this association did not persist for non-Hispanic White women (Heck et al. 1997), suggesting that the long-established positive SES gradient for breast cancer mortality is diminishing for certain advantaged groups. Similar changes in risk patterns have occurred for other diseases such as coronary heart disease, a major cause of morbidity and mortality in the industrialized world. Once considered a disease of the wealthy in the early 1900's, coronary heart disease is now most prevalent among low-income groups (Marmot and Mustard 1994). Although Wilkinson describes hierarchical stress as the primary factor underlying the SES-health association, this mechanism cannot account for the changing risk patterns of disease and death over time.

One way to think about the findings of the resource utilization analyses is in terms of the "web of causation." MacMahon and associates developed the notion of the "web of causation" based upon the belief that the effects of disease evolve due to an interrelated chain of events rather than a single isolated cause (MacMahon and Pugh 1970). In other words, many intersecting antecedent events can develop a situation, which may be thought of as a web. Similarly, resource utilization as described by Link and Phelan in some sense reflects a "web" in that absolute resources act as intersecting facilitating mechanisms to enable one to promote health and reduce risk at the individual, family, or community level.

Although findings suggested that the HRRI captures some aspects of the resource utilization process, this measure was not found to explain the SES-health association. However, results indicate that SES shapes health-related resource utilization, and resource utilization is found to be related to health outcomes as would be predicted by Fundamental Cause theory. The lack of findings suggests two explanations: this operationalization is insufficient to capture the full range of health-related resources, or such resources are not, in fact, the mechanism through which SES is shaping health outcomes. Given that resource utilization is found to be independently and positively associated with SES and better health outcomes, further efforts to operationalize this process are indicated. One approach that might illuminate the many mechanisms through which resources can affect health is an in-depth qualitative study followed by a prospective study to examine resource utilization over a prolonged period of time. Qualitative and historical methods may be better adept at documenting the qualitative differences associated with health-related resources which may, in fact, explain more of the variation in the SES-health association.

104

Implications for Future Research

This study is among a handful of research efforts that directly test the effects of relative deprivation on health outcomes, and the first to directly operationalize the resource utilization process as specified by Fundamental Cause. As such, further research efforts are warranted to specify and refine measures of each of the proposed mediating processes.

Although SES effects on health are thought to be strongest in middle and early old age, social comparison processes such as relative deprivation may be weaker during this life stage. Since financial dissatisfaction and relative deprivation effects have been found to diminish as individuals' age, efforts should be directed at examining relative deprivation within different age groups.

Individuals may compare themselves to others with respect to groups based on a variety of demographic characteristics. Research to explore whether and how demographic-based definitions of reference groups reflect the social comparison process of relative deprivation and its consequent effects on health is an area for further exploration.

Policy Implications

Understanding how SES shapes health outcomes is essential to reducing health disparities throughout the social hierarchy. Empirical findings from this study provide evidence that both material and psychosocial mechanisms underlie the link between socioeconomic status and health. Given that SES is such a robust and persistent predictor of better health and longevity, efforts to examine how public policy serves to limit access to material resources may provide some insight into where public health interventions should be focused. For example, race-based residential segregation, supported through legal, political and economic policy, has been identified as a fundamental determinant of health (Schulz et al. 2002). Schulz and colleagues indicate that race-based residential segregation, typically associated with discriminatory land use zoning and economic divestment, serves to limit educational, employment and housing opportunities. Interventions aimed at changing policy related to zoning regulations may improve access to resources for low and moderate-income families, and thus, may significantly improve the health status of many citizens (Hart et al. 1998). Some suggest that health impact statements be included within all non-health policy proposals (Syme, Lefkowitz, and Krimgold 2002; Link and Phelan 1995).

While studies investigate the mechanisms linking SES to health, efforts could be waged on other fronts. Deaton suggests that efforts be focused on developing health policy which shifts the attention away from health care and health-related behavior to improving education, given its relationship to better health (Deaton 2002). Improving the quality of education as a health intervention is probably an easier case to make within the context of a market-based US economy not easily persuaded to engage in wealth redistribution.

Further investigation to discern how SES shapes health outcomes will inevitably lead to reducing disparities throughout the social hierarchy. Thus, there may be no better way to contribute to improving the nation's health.

References Cited

Adelstein, A. M., "Life-style in occupational cancer," *Journal of Toxicology and Environmental Health* 6: 953-962 (1980).

Adler, Nancy E. et al., "Socioeconomic status and health: the challenge of the gradient," *American Psychologist* 49: 15-24 (1994).

Antonovsky, A., "Social class, life expectancy, and overall mortality," *The Milbank Quarterly* 45: 31-73 (1967).

Baron, Reuben M. and David A. Kenny, "The moderator-mediator variable distinction in social psychological research: conceptual, strategic and statistical considerations," *Journal of Personality and Social Psychology* 51 (6): 1173-1182 (1986).

Bartley, Mel and I. Plewis, "Does health selective social mobility account for socioeconomic differences in health?," *Journal of Health and Social Behavior* 38: 376-386 (1997).

Black, D. et al. 1982. *Inequalities in health: The Black Report.* Edited by P. Townsend and N. Davidson. Middlesex: Penguin.

Blakely, Tony, K. Lochner, and I. Kawachi, "Metropolitan area income inequality and self-rated health--a multi-level study," *Social Science and Medicine* 54: 65-77 (2002).

Buunk, B. P., F. X. Gibbons, and M. Reis-Bergan. 1997. Social comparison in health and illness: a historical overview. In *Health, Coping and Well-Being Perspectives from Social Comparison Theory.* Edited by F. X Gibbons. Mahwah: Lawrence Erlbaum Associates.

Cassel, John, "The contribution of the social environment to host resistance," *American Journal of Epidemiology* 104: 107-123 (1976).

Centers for Disease Control. "Body Mass Index for Adults" At. http://www.cdc.gov/nccdphp/dnpa/bmi/bmi-adult.htm . 2002. 10-21-2002.

Chadwick, Edwin. Report on the sanitary conditions of the labouring population of Great Britain. 1842. Edinburgh, Edinburgh University Press.
Ref Type: Report

Chapin, Charles V., "Deaths among taxpayers and non-taxpayers, income tax, Providence, 1865," *American Journal of Public Health* 14: 647-651 (1924).

Coburn, David and Clyde R. Pope, "Socioeconomic status and preventive health behaviour," *Journal of Health and Social Behavior* 15: 67-78 (1974).

Conley, Dalton. 1999. *Being Black, living in the red: race, wealth and social policy in America.* Berkeley: University of California Press.

Coombs, Lolagene C., "Economic differentials in causes of death," *Medical Care* 1: 246-255 (1941).

Crosby, F. J., "A model of egoistical relative deprivation," *Psychological Review* 83: 85-113 (1976).

Daly, M. C. et al., "Macro-to-micro links in the relation between income inequality and mortality," *Milbank Memorial Fund Quarterly* 76 (3): 315-339 (1998).

Danziger, S. and P. Gottschalk. 1995. *America unequal.* Cambridge: Harvard University Press.

Deaton, A., "Policy implications of the gradient of health and wealth," *Health Affairs* 21 (2): 13-30 (2002).

Diez-Roux, A., B. Link, and M. Northridge, "A multilevel analysis of income inequality and cardiovascular disease risk factors," *Social Science and Medicine* 50: 673-687 (2000).

Diez-Roux, A. et al., "Neighborhood of residence and incidence of coronary heart disease," *New England Journal of Medicine* 345 (2): 99-106 (2001).

Duncan, Greg J., "Income dynamics and health," *International Journal of Health Services* 26: 419-444 (1996).

Duncan, Greg J. and Eric Petersen, "The long and short of asking questions about income, wealth, and labor supply," *Social Science Research* 30: 248-263 (2001).

Eibner, C. E. and Evans, W. N. Relative deprivation, poor health habits, and mortality. http://www.russellsage.org/special_interest/socialinequality/eibner_evans_rsf_inequality_project .pdf . 2001. Working Paper, Russel Sage Foundation.

Eisen, S. A. et al., "Sociodemographic and health status characteristics associated with prostate cancer screening in a national cohort of middle-aged male veterans," *Urology* 53 (3): 516-522 (1999).

Elo, I. T. and S. H. Preston, "Educational differentials in mortality: United States, 1979-85," *Social Science and Medicine* 42: 47-57 (1996).

Elstad, Jon Ivar. 1998. The psycho-social perspective on social inequalities in health. In *The sociology of health inequalities.* Edited by Mel Bartley, David Blane, and G. D. Smith. Oxford: Blackwell Publishers.

Evans, Robert G. 1994. Introduction. In *Why are some people healthy and others not?: the determinants of health of populations.* Edited by Robert G. Evans, M. L. Barer, and Theodore R. Marmor. New York: Aldine de Gruyter.

Feinstein, Jonathan, "The relationship between socioeconomic status and health: a review of the literature," *The Milbank Quarterly* 71 (2): 279-322 (1993).

Finkel, S. E. Causal analysis with panel data. 1995. Thousand Oaks, CA, Sage. Sage University Paper series on Quantitative Applications in the Social Sciences, #07-105. Lewis-Beck, Michael S.

Fiscella, Kevin and Peter Franks, "Poverty or income inequality as a predictor of mortality: longitudinal cohort study," *British Medical Journal* 314: 1724-1727 (1997).

Folger, Robert. 1987. Reformulating the preconditions of resentment: a referent cognitions model. In *Social comparison, social justice and relative deprivation: theoretical, empirical and policy perspectives.* Edited by J. C. Masters and W. P. Smith. Hillsdale, NJ: Lawrence Erlbaum Associates.

Ford, E. S. et al., "Physical activity behaviors in lower and higher socioeconomic status populations," *American Journal of Epidemiology* 133 (12): 1246-1255 (1991).

Ford, Graeme et al., "Patterns of class inequality in health through the lifespan: class gradients at 15, 35, and 55 Years in the west of Scotland," *Social Science and Medicine* 39 (8): 1037-1050 (1994).

GeoLytics, Inc. CensusCD 1990+Maps. (4.0). 1997.

Erica Goode, "For good health, it helps to be rich and important," *The New York Times*, 1999, Science, p. 1.

Gravelle, Hugh, "How much of the relation between population mortality and unequal distribution of income is a statistical artefact?," *British Medical Journal* 316: 382-385 (1998).

Hart, K. D. et al., "Metropolitan governance, residential segregation, and mortality among African-Americans," *American Journal of Public Health* 88 (3): 434-438 (1998).

Hayward, Mark D. et al., "The significance of socioeconomic status in explaining the racial gap in chronic health conditions," *American Sociological Review* 65 (December): 910-930 (2000).

Heck, K. E. et al., "Socioeconomic status and breast cancer mortality, 1989 through 1993: an analysis of education data from death certificates," *American Journal of Public Health* 87 (7): 1218-1222 (1997).

Hill, D. H. 1999. Unfolding bracket method in the measurement of expenditures and wealth. In *Wealth, work and health.* Edited by J. P. Smith and F. T. Juster. Ann Arbor: University of Michigan.

House, James S. et al., "Age, socioeconomic status, and health," *The Milbank Quarterly* 68: 383-411 (1990).

House, James S. et al. 1992. Social stratification, age, and health. In *Aging, Health Behaviors, and Health Outcomes.* Edited by K. Warner Schaie, Dan Blazer, and James S. House. Hillsdale: Lawrence Erlbaum Associates.

House, James S. et al., "The social stratification of aging and health," *Journal of Health and Social Behavior* 35: 213-234 (1994).

Hummer, Robert A., Richard G. Rogers, and Isaac W. Eberstein, "Sociodemographic differentials in adult mortality: review of analytic approaches," *Population and Development Review* 24 (3): 553-578 (1998).

Idler, E. L. and Y. Benyamini, "Self-rated health and mortality: a review of twenty-seven community studies," *Journal of Health and Social Behavior* 38: 21-37 (1997).

IMPUTE: A SAS application system for missing value imputations---with special reference to HRS income/assets imputations Version 3.0. Institute of Social Research.

Jones, L. and M. Sidell. 1997. *The challenge of promoting health.* London: The Open University.

Judd, C. M. and G. H. McClelland. 1989. Simple models: statistical inferences about parameter values. In *Data analysis: a model comparison approach.* New York: Harcourt Brace Jovanovich, Inc.

Judge, Ken, "Income distribution and life expectancy: a critical appraisal," *British Medical Journal* 311: 1282-1285 (1995).

Juster, Thomas and Richard Suzman, "An overview of the Health and Retirement Study," *Journal of Human Resources* 30: S7-S56 (1995).

Kaplan, George et al., "Inequality in income and mortality in the United States: analysis of mortality and potential pathways," *British Medical Journal* 312: 999-1003 (1996).

Karoly, L. 1993. The trend in inequality among families, individuals, and workers in the United States: a twenty-five year perspective. In *Uneven Tides: Rising Inequality in America.* Edited by S. Danziger and P. Gottschalk. New York: Russell Sage.

Katz, M. H. et al., "Impact of socioeconomic status on survival with AIDS," *American Journal of Epidemiology* 148 (3): 282-291 (1998).

Katz, Steven and Timothy P. Hofer, "Socioeconomic disparities in preventive care persist despite universal coverage," *Journal of the American Medical Association* 272 (17): 530-534 (1994).

Kaufman, Jay S. and Richard S. Cooper, "Seeking causal explanations in social epidemiology," *American Journal of Epidemiology* 150 (2): 113-120 (1999).

Kawachi, I. et al., "Social capital, income inequality, and mortality," *American Journal of Public Health* 87: 1491-1499 (1997).

Kenkel, Donald S., "Health behavior, health knowledge, and schooling," *Journal of Political Economy* 99 (2): 287-305 (1991).

Kennedy, B. P., I. Kawachi, and D. Prothrow-Stith, "Income distribution and mortality: cross-sectional ecological study of the Robin Hood index in the United States," *British Medical Journal* 312: 1004-1007 (1996).

Kitagawa, Evelyn M. and P. M. Hauser. 1973. *Differential mortality in the United States: a study in socioeconomic epidemiology.* Cambridge: Harvard University Press.

Krieger, Nancy, David R. Williams, and N. E. Moss, "Measuring social class in US public health research," *Annual Review of Public Health* 18: 341-378 (1997).

Land, K. C. and S. T. Russel, "Wealth accumulation across the adult life course: stability and change in sociodemographic covariate structures of net worth data in the Survey of Income and Program Participation, 1984-1991," *Social Science Research* 25: 423-462 (1996).

Lantz, Paula M. et al., "Socioeconomic factors, health behaviors, and mortality," *Journal of the American Medical Association* 279 (21): 1703-1708 (1998).

Liang, Wenchi et al., "A population-based study of age and gender differences in patterns of health-related behaviors," *American Journal of Preventive Medicine* 17 (1): 8-17 (1999).

Liberatos, Penny, Bruce G. Link, and Jennifer L. Kelsey, "The measurement of social class in epidemiology," *Epidemiologic Reviews* 10: 87-121 (1988).

Lind, E. A. et al., "In the eye of the beholder: Tort litigants' evaluations of their experiences in the civil justice system," *Law and Society Review* 24: 953-996 (1990).

Link, Bruce G. et al., "Social epidemiology and the Fundamental Cause concept: on the structuring of effective cancer screens by socioeconomic status," *The Milbank Quarterly* 76 (3): 375-402 (1998).

Link, Bruce G. and Jo C. Phelan, "Social conditions as fundamental causes of disease," *Journal of Health and Social Behavior* Extra Issue: 80-94 (1995).

Link, Bruce G. and Jo C. Phelan, "Understanding sociodemographic differences in health--the role of fundamental social causes," *American Journal of Public Health* 86 (4): 471-473 (1996).

Link, Bruce G. and Jo C. Phelan. 2000. Evaluating the fundamental cause explanation for social disparities in health. In *Handbook of Medical Sociology.* Fifth ed. Edited by Chloe Bird, Peter Conrad, and Allen Fremont. Upper Saddle River: Prentice Hall.

Lynch, J. et al., "Income inequality and mortality in metropolitan areas in the United States," *American Journal of Public Health* 88: 1074-1080 (1998).

Lynch, John W., "Income inequality and health: expanding the debate," *Social Science and Medicine* 51: 1001-1005 (2000).

Lynch, John W. et al., "Income inequality and mortality: importance to health of individual income, psychosocial environment, or material conditions," *British Medical Journal* 320 (7243): 1200-1204 (2000).

MacMahon, B. and T. F. Pugh. 1970. *Epidemiology principles and methods.* Boston: Little, Brown and Company.

Major, B. and M. Testa, "Social comparison processes and judgments of entitlement and satisfaction," *Journal of Experimental Psychology* 25: 101-120 (1988).

Marmot, M. G. and J. F. Mustard. 1994. Coronary heart disease from a population perspective. In *Why are some people health and others not? The determinants of health of populations.* Edited by Robert G. Evans, M. L. Barer, and Theodore R. Marmor. New York: Aldine De Gruyter.

Marmot, Michael G. et al., "Social inequalities in health : next questions and converging evidence," *Social Science and Medicine* 44 (6): 901-910 (1997).

Marmot, Michael G., Martin Shipley, and Geoffrey Rose, "Inequalities in death--specific explanations of a general pattern?," *The Lancet* 1 (8384): 1003-1006 (1984).

Marmot, Michael G. and R. G. Wilkinson, "Psychosocial and material pathways in the relation between income and health: a response to Lynch et al.," *British Medical Journal* 322: 1233-1236 (2001).

Mellor, Jennifer M. and Jeffrey Milyo, "Reexamining the evidence of an ecological association between income inequality and health," *Journal of Health Politics, Policy and Law* 26 (3): 487-522 (2001).

Menard, S. Longitudinal research. 1991. Newbury Park, CA, Sage. Sage University Paper Series on Quantitative Applications in the Social Sciences, 07-076.

Merton, Robert K. and Alice S. Rossi. 1957. Contributions to the theory of reference group behavior. In *Social theory and social structure: revised and enlarged edition.* Edited by Robert K. Merton. New York: Collier-Macmillan.

Mirowsky, John, "The psycho-economics of feeling underpaid: distributive justice and the earnings of husbands and wives," *American Journal of Sociology* 92 (6): 1404-1434 (1987).

Mirowsky, John. 1999. Analyzing associations between mental health and social circumstances. In *Handbook of the Sociology of Mental Health.* Edited by C. S. Aneshensel and J. C. Phelan. New York: Kluwer Academic/Plenum.

Moon, M. and FT Juster, "Economic status measures in the health and retirement study," *Journal of Human Resources* 30: S138-S157 (1995).

Morris, M. and B. Western, "Inequality in earnings at the close of the twentieth century," *Annual Review of Sociology* 25: 623-657 (1999).

Myers, D. G. 1992. *The pursuit of happiness: who is happy--and why.* New York: Marrow.

Novotny, T. E. et al., "Smoking by Blacks and Whites: socioeconomic and demographic differences," *American Journal of Public Health* 78: 1187-1189 (1988).

Oakes, P. J., S. A. Haslam, and J. C. Turner. 1994. *Stereotyping and social reality.* Oxford, UK: Blackwell.

Omran, A. R., "The epidemiologic transition. a theory of the epidemiology of population change.," *Milbank Memorial Fund Quarterly* 49 (4): 509-538 (1971).

Osborne, Jason W., "Notes on the use of data transformations," *Practical Assessment, Research & Evaluation* 8 (6) (2002).

Paneth, N. and Mervin Susser, "Early origin of coronary heart disease (the "Barker hypothesis")," *British Medical Journal* 310 (6977): 411-412 (1995).

Pappas, G. et al., "The increasing disparity in mortality between socioeconomic groups in the United States, 1960 and 1986," *New England Journal of Medicine* 329: 1522-1526 (1993).

Rindskopf, David, "Linear equality restrictions in regression and loglinear models," *Psychological Bulletin* 96 (3): 597-603 (1984).

Rodgers, G. B., "Income and inequality as determinants or mortality: an international cross-section analysis," *Population Studies* 33: 343-351 (1979).

Rogers, R. G., R. A. Hummer, and C. B. Nam. 2000. *Living and dying in the USA.* New York: Academic Press.

Rogot, E., Paul D. Sorlie, and Norman Johnson, "Life expectancy by employment status, income, and education in the National Longitudinal Mortality Study," *Public Health Reports* 107: 457-461 (1992).

Ross, Catherine E. and John Mirowsky, "Does medical insurance contribute to socioeconomic differentials in health?," *The Milbank Quarterly* 78 (2): 291-321 (2000).

Ross, Catherine E. and Chia-ling Wu, "The links between education and health," *American Sociological Review* 60 (October): 719-745 (1995).

Schieman, S., K. Van Gundy, and J. Taylor, "Status, role, and resource explanations," *Journal of Health and Social Behavior* 42 (March): 80-96 (2001).

Schieman, Scott, "Age, education and the sense of control," *Research on Aging* 23 (2): 153-178 (2001).

Schulz, A. J. et al., "Racial and spatial relations as fundamental determinants of health in Detroit," *The Milbank Quarterly* 80 (4): 677-707 (2002).

Sennett, R and J. Cobb. 1973. *The hidden injuries of class.* New York: Knopf.

Singer, E. 1981. Reference groups and social evaluations. In *Social Psychology: Sociological Perspectives.* Edited by M. Rosenberg and R. H. Turner. New York: Basic Books, Inc.

Soobader, M. J. and F. B. LeClere, "Aggregation and the measurement of income inequality: effects on morbidity," *Social Science and Medicine* 48 (6): 733-744 (1999).

Sorlie, Paul D., E. Backlund, and J. Keller, "US mortality by economic, demographic, and social characteristics: The National Longitudinal Mortality Study," *American Journal of Public Health* 85: 949-956 (1995).

Spilerman, Seymour, "Wealth and stratification processes," *Annual Review of Sociology* 26: 497-524 (2000).

Stata Statistical Software, College Station, TX.

Stouffer, S. A. et al. 1949. *The American soldier: adjustment during army life.* Vol. 1. Princeton: Princeton University Press.

Summers, J. 1989. *Soho -- a history of London's most colourful neighborhood.* London: Bloomsbury.

Susser, Mervin. 1973. *Causal thinking in the health sciences: concepts and strategies in epidemiology.* New York: Oxford University Press.

Susser, Mervyn, William Watson, and Kim Hopper. 1985. *Sociology in medicine.* New York: Oxford University.

Syme, S. L. and L. F. Berkman, "Social Class, susceptibility, and sickness," *American Journal of Epidemiology* 104 (1): 1-8 (1976).

Syme, S. L., Bonnie Lefkowitz, and Barbara K. Krimgold, "Incorporating socioeconomic factors into US health policy: addressing the barriers," *Health Affairs* 21 (2): 113-118 (2002).

Thoits, P. A., "Stress, coping and social support processes--where are we--what next," *Journal of Health and Social Behavior* (Extra Issue): 53-79 (1995).

Tyler, T. R. et al. 1997. *Social justice in a diverse society.* Boulder: Westview Press.

U.S. Department of Health and Human Services. *Healthy People 2010.* 2000. Washington, DC, U.S. Government Printing Office.

Veenstra, G., "Social capital and health (plus wealth, income inequality and regional health governance)," *Social Science and Medicine* 54: 849-868 (2002).

Verbrugge, L. M. and D. L. Wingard, "Sex differentials in health and mortality," *Women and Health* 12 (2): 103-143 (1987).

Waldmann, R. J., "Income distribution and infant mortality," *Quarterly Journal of Economics* 107: 1283-1302 (1992).

Wegener, Bernard, "Relative deprivation and social mobility: structural constraints on distributive justice judgments," *European Sociological Review* 7: 3-18 (1991).

Wilkinson, R. G. 1986a. *Class and health: research and longitudinal data.* London: Tavistock.

Wilkinson, R. G. 1986b. Socio-economic differences in mortality: interpreting the data on their size and trends. In *Class and Health.* Edited by R. G. Wilkinson. London: Tavistock.

Wilkinson, R. G., "Income distribution and life expectancy," *British Medical Journal* 304: 165-168 (1992).

Wilkinson, R. G., "The epidemiological transition: from material scarcity to social disadvantage?," *Daedalus* 123 (61): 77 (1994).

Wilkinson, R. G. 1996. *Unhealthy societies: the afflictions of inequality.* London: Routledge.

Wilkinson, R. G., "Health inequalities: relative or absolute material standards?," *British Medical Journal* 314: 591-595 (1997a).

Wilkinson, R. G., "Income inequality summarizes the health burden of individual relative deprivation," *British Medical Journal* 314 (June 14): 1727-1728 (1997b).

Wilkinson, R. G. 1999. The culture of inequality. In *The society and population health reader: income inequality and health.* Edited by I. Kawachi, B. P. Kennedy, and R. G. Wilkinson. New York: The New Press.

Williams, D. R., "Race, socioeconomic status, and health: the added effects of racism and discrimination," *Annals of the New York Academy of Sciences* 896: 173-188 (1999).

Williams, David R. and Chiquita Collins, "US socioeconomic and racial differences in health: patterns and explanations," *Annual Review of Sociology* 21: 349-386 (1995).

Wilson, Sven E., "Socioeconomic status and the prevalence of health problems among married couples in late midlife," *American Journal of Public Health* 91 (1): 131-135 (2001).

Winkleby, M. A., S. P. Fortmann, and D. C. Barrett, "Social class disparities in risk factors for disease: eight-year prevalence patterns by level of education," *Preventive Medicine* 19: 1-12 (1990).

Wolf, Charlotte, "Relative advantage," *Symbolic Interaction* 13 (1): 37-61 (1990).

Appendix 1

County-level Relative Income Tables

Table A1.1 Relative Income Regression Models among WOMEN; Limited to those with excellent/good health at W1

Linear Regression used for outcome: **Relative Income (County)**   *(n=4,378)*

Covariates	Model 1 Beta (SE)	Model 2 Beta (SE)	Model 3 Beta (SE)	Model 4 Beta (SE)	Model 5 Beta (SE)
Log Household Income	.998† (.008)			1.004† (.007)	1.002† (.007)
Education		.103† (.01)		-.002 (.003)	-.001 (.003)
Log Household Net Worth			1.010† (.099)	-.055** (.020)	-.057* (.022)
Race/ Ethnicity					
White[a]					-.001 (.039)
Hispanic[a]					.031 (.043)
Other[a]					-.011 (.052)
Age					-.001 (.001)
Married[b]					.015 (.015)
R^2	.928	.056	.068	.928	.929

[a] Compared to Blacks;
[b] Compared to never married, divorced, widowed, or separated $p<.05$, **$p<.01$, †$p<.001$

116

Table A1.2 Relative Income Regression Models among MEN; Limited to those with excellent/good health at W1					
Linear Regression used for outcome: **Relative Income (County)** (*n=3,634*)					
Covariates	*Model 1* Beta (SE)	*Model 2* Beta (SE)	*Model 3* Beta (SE)	*Model 4* Beta (SE)	*Model 5* Beta (SE)
Log Household Income	.988† (.007)			.992† (.007)	.989† (.008)
Education		.110† (.005)		.0004 (.002)	.0006 (.003)
Log Household Net Worth			1.023† (.071)	-.039 (.022)	-.039 (.023)
Race/ Ethnicity					
White[a]					-.005 (.036)
Hispanic[a]					-.006 (.040)
Other[a]					.009 (.062)
Age					-.0004 (.002)
Married[b]					.036 (.021)
R^2	.91	.10	.09	.915	.916

[a] Compared to Blacks;
[b] Compared to never married, divorced, widowed, or separated   *p<.05, ** p<.01, † p<.001

117

Covariates	Model 1 Beta (SE)	Model 2 Beta (SE)	Model 3 Beta (SE)	Model 4 Beta (SE)	Model 5 Beta (SE)	Model 6 Beta (SE)	Model 7 Beta (SE)

Table A1.3 Financial Dissatisfaction Coefficients from Explanatory Models (W1-W4) Limited to those with excellent/good health at W1

WOMEN *(n=4,305)*

Covariates	*Model 1* Beta (SE)	*Model 2* Beta (SE)	*Model 3* Beta (SE)	*Model 4* Beta (SE)	*Model 5* Beta (SE)	*Model 6* Beta (SE)	*Model 7* Beta (SE)
Log Income	-.223† (.030)			-.157† (.025)	-.125† (.025)		-.140 (.086)
Education		-.026* (.010)		.019* (.009)	.017 (.010)		.017 (.010)
Log Net Worth			-.026† (.010)	-1.039† (.082)	-.895† (.078)		-.894† (.078
Log Relative Income (County)						-.153† (.026)	.015 (.077)
Race/ Ethnicity							
White [a]					-.198* (.089)	-.306** (.090)	-.198* (.088)
Hispanic [a]					.003 (.127)	-.075 (.135)	.003 (.127)
Other [a]					-.187 (.158)	-.274 (.154)	-.187 (.158)
Age					-.032† (.006)	-.039† (.006)	-.032† (.006)
Married [b]					-.350† .065	-.447† .065	-.350† (.064)

Linear Regression used for outcome: Financial Dissatisfaction
[a] Compared to Blacks;
[b] Compared to never married, divorced, widowed, or separated   *p<.05, **p<.01, † p<.001

118

Table A1.4 Financial Dissatisfaction Coefficients from Explanatory Models (W1-W4) Limited to those with excellent/good health at W1

MEN (n=3,378)

Covariates	Model 1 Beta (SE)	Model 2 Beta (SE)	Model 3 Beta (SE)	Model 4 Beta (SE)	Model 5 Beta (SE)	Model 6 Beta (SE)	Model 7 Beta (SE)
Log Household Income	-.182† (.038)			.020** (.014)	-.113** (.041)		-.072 (.124)
Education		-.011 (.013)		-.113 (.041)	.018 (.014)		.018 (.014)
Log Household Net Worth			-.927† (.127)	-.845† (.155)	-.796† (.143)		-.800† (.143)
Log Relative Income (County)						-.184† (.031)	-.062 (.114)
Race/ Ethnicity							
White [a]					.017 (.141)	-.036 (.138)	.017 (.141)
Hispanic [a]					.105 (.195)	.079 (.185)	.104 (.193)
Other [a]					.148 (.195)	.111 (.192)	.150 (.195)
Age					-.033** .011	-.043** (.013)	-.033** (.011)
Married [b]					.156 (.098)	.136 (.097)	.159 (.098)

Linear Regression used for outcome: Financial Dissatisfaction
[a] Compared to Blacks;
[b] Compared to never married, divorced, widowed, or separated   *p<.05, **p<.01, † p<.001

Table A1.5 Poor Self-Rated Health Status Coefficients from Explanatory Models (W1-W4) Limited to those with excellent/good health at W1

	WOMEN (n=4,378)			
Covariates	Model 1 Beta (SE)	Model 2 Beta (SE)	Model 3 Beta (SE)	Model 4 Beta (SE)
Log	-.195†	-.182†		-.392
Household Income	(.041)	(.039)		(.185)
	-.165†	-.154†		-.154†
Education	(.022)	(.022)		(.022)
Log Household	-.786*	-.587		-.574
Net Worth	(.306)	(.297)		(.297)
Log			-.233†	.209
Relative Income			(.043)	(.181)
(County)				
Race/				
Ethnicity				
White [a]		-.340*	-.508†	-.342*
		(.146)	(.135)	(.144)
Hispanic [a]		.225	.638*	.217
		(.264)	(.255)	(.261)
Other [a]		-.032	-.232	-.032
		(.412)	(.458)	(.410)
Age		-.034*	-.028	-.034*
		(.016)	(.016)	(.016)
Married [b]		-.183	-.215	-.186
		(.137)	(.134)	(.137)

Logistic Regression used for outcome: Poor Self-Rated Health
[a] Compared to Blacks;
[b] Compared to never married, divorced, widowed, or separated *p<.05, **p<.01, †p<.001

| | | MEN (n=3,634) | | |

Table A1.6   Poor Self-Rated Health Status Coefficients from Explanatory Models (W1-W4) Limited to those with excellent/good health at W1

Covariates	Model 1 Beta (SE)	Model 2 Beta (SE)	Model 3 Beta (SE)	Model 4 Beta (SE)
Log	-.233**	-.181**		-.275
Income	(.082)	(.063)		(.215)
Education	-.150†	-.149†		-.149†
	(.020)	(.022)		(.022)
Log	-.593*	-.480		-.475
Net Worth	(.257)	(.245)		(.246)
Log			-.299†	.094
Relative Income			(.073)	(.195)
(County)				
Race/				
Ethnicity				
White [a]		-.464	-.713*	-.465
		(.372)	(.353)	(.371)
Hispanic [a]		-.324	-.009	-.324
		(.459)	(.408)	(.458)
Other [a]		-.140	-.508	-.142
		(.513)	(.480)	(.513)
Age		.005	.013	.005
		(.017)	(.016)	(.017)
Married [b]		-.463*	-.356	-.466*
		(.225)	(.218)	(.228)

Logistic Regression used for outcomes: Poor Self-Rated Health
[a] Compared to Blacks;
[b] Compared to never married, divorced, widowed, or separated *p<.05, **p<.01, †p<.001

Table A1.7   Having Any Life-threatening Conditions Coefficients from Explanatory

Models (W1-W4) Limited to those without any conditions at W1

Covariates	Model 1 Beta (SE)	Model 2 Beta (SE)	Model 3 Beta (SE)	Model 4 Beta (SE)
WOMEN *(n=3,964)*				
Log Household Income	-.119** (.039)	-.106** (.038)		-.191 (.190)
Education	-.069† (.016)	-.073† (.018)		-.073† (.018)
Log Household Net Worth	-.650* (.298)	-.665* (.312)		-.660* (.313)
Log Relative Income (County)			-.150† (.037)	.084 (.195)
Race/ Ethnicity				
White [a]		-.051 (.125)	-.187 (.119)	-.052 (.125)
Hispanic [a]		-.244 (.228)	-.034 (.213)	-.245 (.228)
Other [a]		-.083 (.353)	-.241 (.367)	-.085 (.353)
Age		.030 (.016)	.028 (.017)	.030 (.016)
Married [b]		-.0685919 (.120)	-.113 (.118)	-.070 (.120)

Logistic Regression used for outcomes: Having Any Life-threatening Conditions
[a] Compared to Blacks;
[b] Compared to never married, divorced, widowed, or separated *p<.05, **p<.01, †p<.001

122

Table A1.8	Having Any Life-threatening Conditions Coefficients from Explanatory Models (W1-W4) Limited to those without any conditions at W1			
MEN *(n=3,111)*				
Covariates	*Model 1* Beta (SE)	*Model 2* Beta (SE)	*Model 3* Beta (SE)	*Model 4* Beta (SE)
Log Household Income	-.117* (.048)	-.119* (.049)		.110 (.163)
Education	-.001 (.016)	-.001 (.017)		-.0004 (.017)
Log Household Net Worth	-.253 (.189)	-.366 (.203)		-.379 (.203)
Log Relative Income (County)			-.151** (.049)	-.232 (.160)
Race/ Ethnicity				
White [a]		.001 (.180)	-.030 (.174)	.009 (.178)
Hispanic [a]		-.340 (.263)	-.333 (.262)	-.334 (.263)
Other [a]		-.177 (.455)	-.215 (.449)	-.168 (.453)
Age		.053* (.020)	.049* (.019)	.053* (.020)
Married [b]		.171 (.179)	.169 (.180)	.181 (.181)

Logistic Regression used for outcomes: Having Any Life-threatening Conditions
[a] Compared to Blacks;
[b] Compared to never married, divorced, widowed, or separated   *p<.05, **p<.01, †p<.001

Table A1.9 Mortality Coefficients from Explanatory Models (W1-W4)				
Women (n=6,582)				
Covariates	*Model 1* Beta (SE)	*Model 2* Beta (SE)	*Model 3* Beta (SE)	*Model 4* Beta (SE)
Log Household Income	-.267† (.072)	-.210* (.092)		-.116 (.264)
Education	-.040 (.021)	-.047 (.023)		-.048* (.023)
Log Household Net Worth	-1.252* (.581)	-1.240* (.562)		-1.253* (.562)
Log Relative Income (County)			-.298† (.076)	-.096 (.254)
Race/ Ethnicity				
White [a]		-.391* (.171)	-.534** (.172)	-.390* (.171)
Hispanic [a]		-.780** (.241)	-.648** (.227)	-.782** (.240)
Other [a]		.153 (.343)	.062 (.339)	.156 (.343)
Age		.070* (.031)	.066* (.031)	.069* (.031)
Married [b]		-.109 (.188)	-.176 (.201)	-.104 (.189)
Logistic Regression used for outcomes: All-Cause Mortality [a] Compared to Blacks; [b] Compared to never married, divorced, widowed, or separated $*p<.05, **p<.01, †p<.001$				

Table A1.10 Mortality Coefficients from Explanatory Models (W1-W4)				
Men (n=5,731)				
Covariates	Model 1 Beta (SE)	Model 2 Beta (SE)	Model 3 Beta (SE)	Model 4 Beta (SE)
Log Household Income	-.463† (.074)	-.408† (.077)		-.481 (.246)
Education	-.016 (.023)	-.025 (.025)		-.024 (.024)
Log Household Net Worth	-.249 (.329)	-.392* (.359)		-.386 (.360)
Log Relative Income (County)			-.449† (.071)	.076 (.247)
Race/ Ethnicity				
White [a]		-.246 (.203)	-.343 (.209)	-.246 (.203)
Hispanic [a]		-1.135** (.362)	-1.058** (.347)	-1.136** (.363)
Other [a]		-.047 (.542)	-.179 (.564)	-.042 (.537)
Age		.093† (.016)	.093† (.016)	.092† (.016)
Married [b]		-.147 (.173)	-.161 (.176)	-.148 (.173)

Logistic Regression used for outcomes: Having Any Life-threatening Conditions
[a] Compared to Blacks;
[b] Compared to never married, divorced, widowed, or separated *p<.05, **p<.01, †p<.001

Appendix 2

State-level Relative Income Tables

Table A2.1	Relative Income Regression Models among WOMEN; Limited to those with excellent/good health at W1				
Linear Regression used for outcome: **Relative Income (State)**					*(n=4,378)*
Covariates	Model 1 Beta (SE)	Model 2 Beta (SE)	Model 3 Beta (SE)	Model 4 Beta (SE)	Model 5 Beta (SE)
Log Income	.984† (.004)			.990† (.004)	.986† (.004)
Education		.100† (.009)		-.004* (.002)	-.004* (.002)
Log Net Worth			1.002† (.096)	-.046** (.013)	-.055† (.014)
Race/ Ethnicity					
White[a]					.021 (.013)
Hispanic[a]					-.044* (.020)
Other[a]					-.032 (.023)
Age					-.0001 (.001)
Married[b]					.027* (.011)
R^2	.97†	.06†	.07†	.98†	.98†
Linear Regression used for outcome: Relative Income [a] Compared to Blacks; [b] Compared to never married, divorced, widowed, or separated *p<.05,**p<.01,†p<.001					

126

	Model 1 Beta (SE)	Model 2 Beta (SE)	Model 3 Beta (SE)	Model 4 Beta (SE)	Model 5 Beta (SE)

**Table A2.2 Relative Income Regression Models among MEN;
Limited to those with excellent/good health at W1**

Linear Regression used for outcome: **Relative Income (State)** _(n=3,634)_

Covariates	Model 1 Beta (SE)	Model 2 Beta (SE)	Model 3 Beta (SE)	Model 4 Beta (SE)	Model 5 Beta (SE)
Log Income	.977† (.006)			.984† (.005)	.979† (.005)
Education		.106† (.005)		-.003* (.001)	-.004** (.001)
Log Net Worth			1.006† (.079)	-.042** (.012)	-.049† (.012)
Race/ Ethnicity					
White[a]					.041* (.018)
Hispanic[a]					-.046* (.022)
Other[a]					-.016 (.031)
Age					.0003 (.001)
Married[b]					.046** (.017)
R^2	.97†	.10†	.10†	.97†	.97†

Linear Regression used for outcome: Relative Income
[a] Compared to Blacks;
[b] Compared to never married, divorced, widowed, or separated   *p<.05, ** p<.01, † p<.001

Table A2.3 Financial Dissatisfaction Coefficients from Explanatory Models (W1-W4) Limited to those with excellent/good health at W1)

WOMEN (n=4,305)

Covariates	Model 1 Beta (SE)	Model 2 Beta (SE)	Model 3 Beta (SE)	Model 4 Beta (SE)	Model 5 Beta (SE)	Model 6 Beta (SE)	Model 7 Beta (SE)
Log Income	-.223† (.030)			-.157† (.026)	-.125† (.026)		.174 (.108)
Education		.026* (.011)		.020* (.010)	.017 (.011)		.015 (.010)
Log Net Worth			-1.164† (.083)	-1.039† (.082)	-.895† (.078)		-.911† (.079)
Log Relative Income (State)						-.174† (.030)	-.303** (112)
Race/ Ethnicity							
White [a]					-.198* (.089)	-.297** (.091)	-.192* (.090)
Hispanic [a]					.003 (.127)	-.085 (.136)	-.010 (.130)
Other [a]					-.187 (.158)	-.274 (.155)	-.198 (.161)
Age					-.032† (.007)	-.039† (.007)	-.032† (.007)
Married [b]					-.350† (.065)	-.432† (.066)	-.342† (.066)

Linear Regression used for outcome: Financial Dissatisfaction
[a] Compared to Blacks;
[b] Compared to never married, divorced, widowed, or separated   *p<.05, **p<.01, † p<.001

Table A2.4 Financial Dissatisfaction Coefficients from Explanatory Models (W1-W4) Limited to those with excellent/good health at W1

			MEN (n=3,378)				
Covariates	Model 1 Beta (SE)	Model 2 Beta (SE)	Model 3 Beta (SE)	Model 4 Beta (SE)	Model 5 Beta (SE)	Model 6 Beta (SE)	Model 7 Beta (SE)
Log Income	-.182† (.038)			-.113** (.042)	-.134** (.038)		.205 (.148)
Education		-.012 (.014)		.020 (.015)	.019 (.015)		.017 (.015)
Log Net Worth			-.928† (.127)	-.845† (.156)	-.797† (.144)		-.814† (.142)
Log Relative Income (State)						-.204† (.038)	-.345* (.157)
Race/ Ethnicity							
White [a]					.017 (.142)	-.201 (.143)	.031 (.143)
Hispanic [a]					.106 (.195)	.075 (.191)	.091 (.201)
Other [a]					.148 (.195)	.109 (.195)	.140 (.200)
Age					-.034** (.011)	-.044** (.014)	-.034** (.011)
Married [b]					.156 (.098)	.151 (.096)	.172 (.096)

Linear Regression used for outcome: Financial Dissatisfaction
[a] Compared to Blacks;
[b] Compared to never married, divorced, widowed, or separated   *p<.05, **p<.01, † p<.001

Table A2.5 Poor Self-Rated Health Status Coefficients from Explanatory Models

(W1-W4) Limited to those with excellent/good health at W1

WOMEN *(n=4,378)*

Covariates	Model 1 Beta (SE)	Model 2 Beta (SE)	Model 3 Beta (SE)	Model 4 Beta (SE)
Log	-.196†	-.182†		-.273
Income	(.041)	(.040)		(.317)
Education	-.165†	-.154†		-.154†
	(.022)	(.023)		(.023)
Log	-.786*	-.587		-.580
Net Worth	(.306)	(.297)		(.298)
Log			-.254†	.092
Relative			(.048)	(.323)
Income				
(State)				
Race/				
Ethnicity				
White [a]		-.340*	-.499†	-.342*
		(.146)	(.135)	(.145)
Hispanic [a]		.225	.621*	.230
		(.264)	(.255)	(.270)
Other [a]		-.031	-.235	-.031
		(.412)	(.460)	(.412)
Age		-.034*	-.028	-.035*
		(.016)	(.017)	(.016)
Married [b]		-.183	-.202	-.186
		(.137)	(.136)	(.138)

Logistic Regression used for outcome: Self-Rated Health
[a] Compared to Blacks;
[b] Compared to never married, divorced, widowed, or separate *p<.05, **p<.01, †p<.001

Table A2.6 Poor Self-Rated Health Status Coefficients from Explanatory Models (W1-W4) Limited to those with excellent/good health at W1

	MEN (n=3,634)			
Covariates	Model 1 Beta (SE)	Model 2 Beta (SE)	Model 3 Beta (SE)	Model 4 Beta (SE)
Log Income	-.233** (.082)	-.182** (.063)		.110 (.395)
Education	-.150† (.020)	-.150† (.022)		-.151† (.022)
Log Net Worth	-.594* (.257)	-.481 (.246)		-.501* (.249)
Log Relative Income (State)			-.329** (.091)	-.297 (.403)
Race/ Ethnicity				
White [a]		-.465 (.372)	-.690* (.340)	-.452 (.360)
Hispanic [a]		-.325 (.460)	-.021 (.401)	-.339 (.465)
Other [a]		-.140 (.513)	-.509 (.479)	-.141 (.514)
Age		.005 (.017)	.013 (.017)	.005 (.018)
Married [b]		-.463* (.226)	-.332 (.211)	-.449* (.221)

Logistic Regression used for outcomes: Self-Rated Health
[a] Compared to Blacks;
[b] Compared to never married, divorced, widowed, or separated   *p<.05, **p<.01,
†p<.001

131

Table A2.7 Having Any Life-threatening Conditions Coefficients from Explanatory

Models (W1-W4) Limited to those without any conditions at W1

Covariates	Model 1 Beta (SE)	Model 2 Beta (SE)	Model 3 Beta (SE)	Model 4 Beta (SE)
WOMEN *(n=3,964)*				
Log Income	-.120** (.040)	-.107** (.039)		-.268 (.339)
Education	-.069† (.016)	-.073† (.019)		-.072† (.018)
Log Net Worth	-.651* (.298)	-.665* (.312)		-.653* (.314)
Log Relative Income (State)			-.158† (.033)	.163 (.333)
Race/ Ethnicity				
White [a]		.052 (.126)	-.185 (.120)	-.054 (.126)
Hispanic [a]		-.245 (.228)	-.042 (.215)	-.235 (.225)
Other [a]		-.084 (.354)	-.248 (.368)	-.078 (.353)
Age		.030 (.017)	.028 (.017)	.030 (.016)
Married [b]		-.069 (.120)	-.107 (.118)	-.073 (.119)

Logistic Regression used for outcomes: Having Any Life-threatening Conditions
[a] Compared to Blacks;
[b] Compared to never married, divorced, widowed, or separated *p<.05, **p<.01, †p<.001

132

Table A2.8 Having Any Life-threatening Conditions Coefficients from Explanatory Models (W1-W4) Limited to those without any conditions at W1

MEN *(n=3,111)*

Covariates	Model 1 Beta (SE)	Model 2 Beta (SE)	Model 3 Beta (SE)	Model 4 Beta (SE)
Log Income	-.118* (.048)	-.120* (.050)		-.190 (.339)
Education	-.001 (.016)	.001 (.017)		-.0004 (.017)
Log Net Worth	-.253 (.189)	-.366 (.203)		-.363 (.200)
Log Relative Income (State)			-.142** (.048)	.072 (.339)
Race/ Ethnicity				
White [a]		.002 (.180)	-.039 (.175)	.001 (.179)
Hispanic [a]		-.340 (.264)	-.344 (.264)	-.335 (.263)
Other [a]		-.178 (.456)	-.241 (.452)	-.173 (.457)
Age		.053* (.020)	.050* (.019)	.053* (.020)
Married [b]		.171 (.180)	.157 (.180)	.168 (.181)

Logistic Regression used for outcomes: Having Any Life-threatening Conditions
[a] Compared to Blacks;
[b] Compared to never married, divorced, widowed, or separated   *p<.05, **p<.01, †p<.001

133

Table A2.9 Mortality Coefficients from Explanatory Models (W1-W4)

		Women (n=6,582)		
Covariates	*Model 1* Beta (SE)	*Model 2* Beta (SE)	*Model 3* Beta (SE)	*Model 4* Beta (SE)
Log Income	-.267† (.072)	-.210* (.092)		.109 (.519)
Education	-.040 (.021)	-.047 (.023)		-.048* (.024)
Log Net Worth	-1.252* (.581)	-1.240* (.562)		-1.267* (.566)
Log Relative Income (State)			-.313† (.075)	-.324 (.506)
Race/ Ethnicity				
White [a]		-.391* (.171)	-.514** (.174)	-.382* (.177)
Hispanic [a]		-.780** (.241)	-.673** (.229)	-.800** (.242)
Other [a]		.153 (.343)	.073 (.338)	.157 (.343)
Age		.070* (.031)	.065* (.031)	.069* (.031)
Married [b]		-.109 (.188)	-.164 (.197)	-.100 (.184)

Logistic Regression used for outcomes: All-Cause Mortality
[a] Compared to Blacks;
[b] Compared to never married, divorced, widowed, or separated   *p<.05, **p<.01, †p<.001

134

Table A2.10 Mortality Coefficients from Explanatory Models (W1-W4)

Men (n=5,731)

Covariates	Model 1 Beta (SE)	Model 2 Beta (SE)	Model 3 Beta (SE)	Model 4 Beta (SE)
Log Income	-.463† (.074)	-.408† (.077)		-.535 (.316)
Education	-.016 (.023)	-.025 (.025)		-.024 (.024)
Log Net Worth	-.249 (.329)	-.392* (.359)		-.385 (.360)
Log Relative Income (State)			-.457† (.070)	.129 (.317)
Race/ Ethnicity				
White [a]		-.246 (.203)	-.322 (.208)	-.248 (.206)
Hispanic [a]		-1.135** (.362)	-1.104** (.349)	-1.126** (.358)
Other [a]		-.047 (.542)	-.155 (.561)	-.041 (.534)
Age		.093† (.016)	.091† (.016)	.093† (.016)
Married [b]		-.147 (.173)	-.141 (.175)	-.150 (.172)

Logistic Regression used for outcomes: Having Any Life-threatening Conditions
[a] Compared to Blacks;
[b] Compared to never married, divorced, widowed, or separated   *p<.05, **p<.01, †p<.001

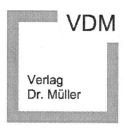